AN ETHNOGRAPHY OF A CHIROPRACTIC CLINIC

Definitions of a Deviant Situation

by James B. Cowie
and Julian Roebuck

THE FREE PRESS
A Division of Macmillan Publishing Co., Inc.
NEW YORK

Collier Macmillan Publishers
LONDON

To James and Elizabeth Cowie
with love and respect

Copyright © 1975 by The Free Press
A Division of Macmillan Publishing Co., Inc.

The Free Press
A Division of Macmillan Publishing Co., Inc.
866 Third Avenue, New York, N.Y. 10022

Collier Macmillan Canada, Ltd.

Library of Congress Catalog Card Number: 75–2811

Printed in the United States of America

printing number

1   2   3   4   5   6   7   8   9   10

Library of Congress Cataloging in Publication Data

Cowie, James B
    An ethnography of a chiropractic clinic.

    Bibliography: p.
    Includes index.
    1. Chiropractic--Social aspects. 2. Chiropractic
clinics. I. Roebuck, Julian, joint author. II. Title.
[DNLM: 1. Chiropractic. 2. Ethnology. 3. Social
behavior. WB905 C741e]
RZ242.C68   615'.534   75-2811
ISBN 0-02-906730-8

Copyright Acknowledgment

Quotes from *Five Years of Articles on Practice Building and Office Procedure* by James W. Parker (Fort Worth, Texas: Share International, 1965) reprinted by permission of The Parker Chiropractic Research Foundation.

"The Thirty-Three Principles of Chiropractic Philosophy" (pp. xxxi–xxxiii) and other quotes (pp. 336–337) from *Chiropractic Textbook* by Ralph W. Stephenson (Davenport, Iowa: Palmer College of Chiropractic, 1948) reprinted by permission of the publisher.

Quotes from "Social Strain and Social Adjustment in the Marginal Role of the Chiropractor," an unpublished doctoral dissertation by Walter I. Wardwell, used by permission of the author.

iii

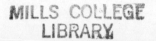

Contents

Preface

The "Chicago school" of thought referred to as symbolic interactionism is universally recognized as a major force in the theoretical tradition of American sociology. Yet, one of the most common criticisms leveled at the interactionist perspective is its alleged inability to come to grips with the "absurd" complexity of social reality which its adherents insist must be taken into account. Thus, the approach has been criticized—often justifiably—for a lack of coherence.

The original study of the social behavior occurring within a chiropractic clinic which ultimately led to the writing of this book was undertaken with the express purpose of trying to coherently reconstruct situationally limited social phenomena while intentionally keeping to the basic premises of symbolic interactionism. We have set forth neither any major new point of view nor a minor theoretical twist in our interactionist approach. Rather, the attempt has been made to devise a situationally heuristic methodology which would meet the demands imposed by the subject matter at hand, remain faithful to the underlying premises of the interactionist tradition, and contribute to the rapidly growing interest in the sociology of everyday life.

We have observed in our classes students who, quite obviously, have experienced the excitement which comes from discovering the novelty and impact of the interactionist approach. Most students however, at some time in their intellectual growth, express some doubts concerning the direct and cogent application of this set of ideas to the study of specific social phenomena. Indeed, much of the literature supporting the interactionist approach seeks—almost apologetically—to explain away this dearth of systematic interactional analysis. It is hoped that the present work will be helpful to those who seek reinforcement in their belief that symbolic interactionism does have the potential for solid methodological explication.

A work of this nature should appeal to a wide variety of interests in the social sciences. The current interest in the dramaturgy of everyday life has led to a focus upon spacially and temporally limited behavior settings. A major section in the book is devoted to a clarification of this concept. Students in sociological research methods courses almost invariably express interest in a methodology of this type due primarily to its appeal as a readily applicable technique. Specifically, students of the labeling approach to deviant behavior should find the present means of analysis useful in a variety of contexts. Further, it should appeal to many general sociologists who have specialized areas of teaching interest—for example, the sociology of occupations, medical sociology, dramaturgical sociology, and the sociology of religion. Finally, we have been encouraged by anthropologists who insist that what is needed in that field are more examples of the application of traditional field techniques to contemporary social situations.

Writing for a diverse audience is not an easy task. Yet, the subject of chiropractic in general has an almost immediate appeal even to those persons only vaguely knowledgeable of this unique form of health care practice. As will be seen, chiropractic is a fascinating and controversial subject, full of curiosities, ambiguities, even mysteries in the classical sense. The present study, however, is not devoted to the study of chiropractic as such. It is concerned with presenting an ethnographic portrait of one chiropractic clinic in one section of the United States and should not be construed as being representational of the entire chiropractic profession.

Basing our opinion on personal experience and a close reading of the literature available, we wish to make it clear that we feel that chiropractic in general has been subject to much unfounded and uninformed criticism. On the other hand, it is not our intention to support or otherwise condone any claims put forth by individual chiropractors or the chiropractic profession in general. On the contrary, we the authors, not being qualified protectors of the public health, must state clearly at the outset that it is impossible for us to come to any empirically supportable conclusions concerning the long-term physiological consequences of chiropractic treatment, *one way or another*. We would like to add, however, that in our experience most qualified practitioners of chiropractic are honest, dedicated, and conscientious men and women, seriously concerned with the health of their patients. There are, of course, exceptions, as in any public service profession. However, due primarily to the passage of chiropractic licensing laws in most of the United States, there has been a decline in the number of untrained persons who call themselves chiropractors for the sole purpose of duping the public.

The practitioner in the clinic in this study was well trained in his profession and demonstrated great skill in its techniques. Moreover, he was a humanitarian in that he envisioned a better world if all people could "experience the benefits of spinal adjustment." The observations reported in this book are in no way intended to cast dispersions or doubts upon him or others in his profession. We have tried to be as honest and precise in our reporting as is humanly possible.

Perhaps a note concerning the authors' joint efforts in this undertaking is appropriate. This project was originally conceived and planned by us some time in advance of the actual data-gathering in the clinic. Many hours were spent in a careful search for every scrap of information concerning chiropractic and a methodology appropriate to the kinds of questions we were prepared to ask. The first person singular is used throughout the text for the following reasons: (1) the senior author, the participant observer (member participant) in the clinic, recorded in the first person the observations upon which the reconstruction of the setting is based; (2) the personal pronoun "I" serves a stylistic purpose in that it obviates the necessity of several referential pronouns. All of the material contained herein was carefully, sometimes painstakingly, reviewed by us both at the end of each day of observation.

There is an advantage to having one member of the research team remain "on the outside," in that he serves as a ready audience for the data as it is gathered and arranged for presentation. Many times, questions which should have been obvious to the participant observer had been overlooked due to his immediate and personal involvement with his subject matter. Once these omissions or inconsistencies were brought to focus, they served as general guidelines for subsequent observations and were duly recorded in the fieldnotes.

Acknowledgments

We wish to express our thanks first and foremost to the chiropractor about whom this study is written, to his wife, and to his many patients who consented to assist in our investigation. However, since it is not the purpose of this book to publicize any of these persons, their names, identities, and residences have been disguised. For the purpose of readability, we have used fictional initials or fictional first names in referring to these persons.

We have unashamedly made use of the conceptual framework of Erving Goffman. Without his pioneer work in the sociology of everyday drama, this book could not have been written in its present form.

Our thanks also to Troy Duster, Wolfgang Frese, Mohamed El-Attar, Louise M. Robbins, and Jack Headblom, who read earlier drafts of the manuscript and offered many helpful comments.

The Free Press editorial staff were most cooperative; our

special thanks to Assistant Vice-President Charles E. Smith and to our project editor, George A. Rowland, for their encouragement, suggestions, and cooperation.

Finally, our heartfelt appreciation goes to our spouses, Marla and Elizabeth, whose support proved to be in a very real sense the backbone of this project.

CHAPTER ONE

Introduction to an Ethnographic Analysis of a Chiropractic Clinic

The following is an ethnographic analysis of a chiropractic clinic primarily from the points of view and social meanings of those actors in this behavior setting: the chiropractor himself, his full-time assistant, and a wide representation of his patients. As will be demonstrated, the chiropractor, although his profession is now legal (licensed) in every state, continues to endure a deviant status in American society. Such marginal deviance demands careful analysis by sociologists.

This study is unique in that the limited research done on the chiropractor has yielded data gathered from an assumed objective stance. Furthermore, the methodology employed hopefully will add to our understanding of the chiropractor and other marginally deviant social positions.

Traditionally, part of the subject matter of ethnographers has been the study of native theories of illness and healing practices. As McCorkle (1961) has pointed out, "growing interest in the field of culture and medical care has led to intensive work on the nature and meaning of folk medicine." Deviant, non-Western medical theories and practices persist in some populations in the United States, including upper middle-class Americans, usually in the form of spurious nostrums, devices, and treatments (Roebuck and Hunter, 1972). The question has been raised as to whether or not these competing systems actually satisfy patient needs which are incompletely fulfilled by the medical establishment (McCorkle, Ibid.).

Many contemporary students of deviance (Rubington and Weinberg, 1973), are beginning to recognize the value of studying the phenomenon of deviant behavior in more conventional contexts (e.g., the "establishment" physician, the physically handicapped, the institutionalized mentally ill, and the dying patient) in contrast with the classical foci upon the obviously outcast (e.g., delinquents or drug addicts).

The most influential of the competing health care systems in the United States is chiropractic. Chiropractic rejects the germ theory of disease—the contemporary view held by Western medical scientists that most illnesses have as their cause some variety of microorganism—and replaces it with a fundamentally unique concept (spinal malallignment) of the cause of all illness. This health care system began in 1895 in Davenport, Iowa, and since then has become firmly established in this country. Its practitioners are trained in chiropractic colleges and are joined together as members of several organizations. In this sense it may be considered an organized discipline.

Although chiropractors represent the largest organized body of marginal health practitioners in the United States (13,729 listed in the 1970 census), little systematic study of this form of health care has been undertaken. Leis (1971), in an attempt to generalize to the professionalism of various occupational groups, examined the emergence of chiropractic as a professional organization. Drawing a sample of 178 New York State chiropractors, Leis tested eight hypotheses, all of which were designed to objectively measure their professional characteristics. Focusing upon the division in the chiropractic profession (discussed in Chapter Two below), this study also sought to examine the problem of loyalty in this profession since the chiropractor must pledge allegience to one of the two competing philosophical camps.

Sternberg (1969), through the use of direct observation, interviews, and lengthy questionnaires, sought to examine the socialization of students attending chiropractic colleges. Evidence which documented the internalization of the stigma attached to chiropractic by society was presented. The stigma was shown to be a central feature in the chiropractic subculture at these colleges.

Both of the studies cited above have attempted to generalize from chiropractic as a profession to professionalism trans-situationally. Very little work, on the other hand, has been done on the chiropractor at work; the main exception is the initial systematic examination of chiropractic by Wardwell (1951). In Wardwell's *Social Strain and Social Adjustment in the Marginal Role of the Chiropractor*, a Parsonian functional approach was employed to analyze the general phenomenon of strain reduction in the larger social structure. Here again, however, the goal was to generalize about the profession as a whole and even beyond to similar marginal roles.

Prior to the publication of that study, no study of the chiropractor in his natural setting had been made. The objective of the present work is to add to our information.

LABELING THE CHIROPRACTOR AS DEVIANT

As Roebuck and Hunter have indicated, contemporary students of deviant behavior "stress the importance of labeling and sanctioning processes and social roles in determining who or what is deviant (1970)." Deviant behavior is behavior that people so label (Becker, 1963). Roebuck (1970) has designated five formal, rule-making, labeling, and sanctioning bodies within the health care area: (1) the American Medical Association, (2) federal agencies, (3) the scientific establishment, (4) commercial associations, and (5) state agencies. The following extracts have been selected from public statements made by representatives of the labeling bodies. The American Medical Association in a statement on chiropractic adopted by AMA House of Delegates:

It is the position of the medical profession that chiropractic is an unscientific cult whose practitioners lack the necessary training and background to diagnose and treat human disease. Chiropractic constitutes a hazard to rational health care in the

United States because of the substandard and unscientific education of its practitioners and their rigid adherence to an irrational, unscientific approach to disease causation. [1966]

The U. S. Department of Health, Education, and Welfare submitted to Congress the following conclusion concerning chiropractic:

There is a body of basic scientific knowledge related to health, disease, and health care. Chiropractic practitioners ignore or take exception to much of this knowledge despite the fact that they have not undertaken adequate scientific research. . . . The inadequacies of chiropractic education, coupled with a theory that de-emphasizes proven causative factors in disease processes, proven methods of treatment, and differential diagnosis, make it unlikely that a chiropractor can make an adequate diagnosis and know the appropriate treatment. . . . [W. J. Cohen, Secretary of HEW, 1968]

The Scientific Establishment—Lindesmith (1968), commenting upon an article by McCorkle (1961) which objectively dealt with the chiropractic in rural Iowa, has pointed out that

even this sympathetic anthropologist thinks of chiropractic as a "deviant theory of disease and treatment"—using modern medicine as his baseline of comparison. . . . Likewise, in a recent book of readings in the *Sociology of Medical Institutions* (1966), a section is entitled "Marginal Healers." The editors assume that there will be the eventual triumph of scientific medicine [over chiropractic]."[1]

[1] It is ironic that even Roebuck and Hunter, who have delineated the labeling bodies discussed in this section, have contributed to the deviant image of chiropractic by publishing an article which designates it as such to a scientific reading public.

The Consumer Federation of America, representing 184 local, state, and national consumer-oriented organizations with millions of members throughout the nation, is concerned

that studies of chiropractics [sic] have not produced evidence of the scientific validity of chiropractic theory and practices, [and] . . . is gravely concerned that chiropractic services would needlessly expose [patients] to potential health hazards. [CFA Resolution, adopted August 29, 1970]

The Medical Society of the State of New York:

Chiropractic is an unscientific cult whose practitioners lack the necessary training and background to diagnose and treat human disease, which is the practice of medicine. . . . Medicine, the allied professions, the voluntary health agencies, and informed people everywhere must be united to thwart the efforts of a common enemy whenever and wherever it rears its ugly head. Against the quack, our best defense is an attack." [H. I. Fineberg, M.D., 1968]

To Roebuck's five formal sanctioning bodies a sixth category could be added: Private interest groups. AFL–CIO:

Care of patients should only be entrusted to those who have a sound scientific knowledge of disease and whose experience and competence render them capable of diagnosing and treating patients by utilizing all the resources of modern medicine. Since neither chiropractic theory nor the quality of chiropractic education equip chiropractors to do this, the AFL–CIO opposes . . .

chiropractic. [A. J. Biemiller, Director, AFL–CIO Legislative Department, 1970]

The National Council of Senior Citizens:

Chiropractic treatment, designed to eliminate causes that do not exist while denying the existence of the real causes, is at best worthless—and at worst mortally dangerous. [*Senior Citizen News,* 1969]

The above public statements made by persuasive labeling groups illustrate that chiropractors endure a deviant or at least marginal role in the United States today. As Roebuck (1970) has noted, these powerful sanctioning organizations operate at different levels in the social order, affecting various segments of the population. Furthermore, not all of these formal groups agree upon common definitions nor do they present to the public a unified and consistent view of chiropractic. It is obvious that some persons and groups reject the deviant label and/or the affixed sanction imposed by these bodies.

The recent interest in medical sociology has generated a need for additional knowledge about limited, marginal, and quasi-practitioners of various kinds. In addition, there seems to be a growing interest in the powerful institutions—for instance, the American Medical Association—as labelers of deviant roles (in this case, that of the chiropractor). This type of inquiry is reflected in the work of Wardwell (1955), McCorkle (1961), Lindesmith and Strauss (1968), and others.

ORIENTATION OF THE STUDY

Ball, in his often cited *Ethnography of an Abortion Clinic* (1967), notes that the study of deviant behavior has long suffered from a lack of primary data. Most analyses depend upon data gathered from the actual social phenomena. Both of the official statistics[2] and the self-reports by participants removed from the theater of action do not represent an unbiased sample of actors, actions, or social organization. Techniques similar to those advocated by Goffman (1959), Becker and Geer (1960), Cavan (1966), Blumer (1969), Denzin (1970), Ball (1967; 1973), and Roebuck and Frese (forthcoming) represent an alternative method to the study of deviance. Ball proposes that we go "directly to the unconventional actors and their subcultures; it is only with such procedures that the natural context of deviance can be studied without the skewedness typical of the usual sources of data." (Ball, ibid.: 295)

This type of research endeavor is a direct outgrowth of the Chicago school of symbolic interactionism as it was set forth primarily in the work of George Herbert Mead (1932, 1936, 1938, and esp. 1943). It is not necessary to review extensively the entire history and range of this approach. Herbert Blumer, in his excellent work *Symbolic Interaction* (1969), has summarized the three premises of symbolic interaction:

---

[2] For an excellent discussion of the limitations of official statistics as a data source, see Douglas (1971).

. . . human beings act toward things on the basis of meanings
that the things have for them. Such things include everything
that the human being may note in his world . . . .

. . . the meaning of such things is derived from, or arises out of,
the social interaction that one has with one's fellows.

. . . these meanings are handled in, and modified through, an
interpretative process used by the persons in dealing with the
things he encounters. [Ibid.:2]

   In light of these principles, the present study is specifically concerned with a description of the practices exhibited
by all actors in a chiropractic behavior setting (hereafter referred to as the Clinic) which exemplify their definitions of
that situation. It is assumed that these actors—both patients
and staff—have *social definitions* of the situation which are
evidenced by their conduct (premise 1). Consequently, in
the present study it is assumed that these actors create and
maintain *rationalizations* for their conduct in order to make
that conduct presentable to themselves and to others (premise 2).[3] They present to themselves, as well as to others, a
construction of the behavior setting through their *actions*
(premise 3). Thus, the main concern of this study will be
an analysis of a chiropractic clinic defined in terms of the
interactional patterns characteristic of that behavior setting.

   [3]The assumption is based upon Mead's concept of self, which implies
that the human being has the capacity to respond not only to the
gestures of others but to his own. In referring to the human being as
having a self, Mead means that the actor in any setting may act socially
toward himself as well as toward others. For a concise summary of this
process, see Meltzer, 1959:15–18.

THE METHODOLOGY OF SYMBOLIC INTERACTIONISM

Denzin, in his book *The Research Act* (1970), has out-lined a series of methodological principles which are re-quired by the interactionist perspective. Among these, sev-eral are especially relevant for present purposes.[4]

First, the symbolic nature (definitions) of social situa-tions and the interaction taking place within them must be considered together if the investigation is to be complete. Other research methods, such as the exclusive use of ques-tionnaires and attitude surveys, fail to capture the emergent and novel aspects of human behavior.

Second, if the reflective nature of self—the process of analyzing one's own being—is to be captured, the re-searcher must assume the standpoint of each actor in the ongoing social situation and view the role-taking process as engaged in by each of those actors.

Furthermore, when the investigator links the definitions of situations and the self definitions of actors within those situations, both must be viewed as relative to those social relationships which furnish him with those symbols and conceptions. Closely associated with this principle is the observation that society provides for its members a variety of behavior settings within which various behaviors occur. Interactional methodology must, therefore, take into ac-count these situated aspects of human behavior. Moreover,

[4] For a complete discussion of these principles, see Denzin, 1970: 7–29. Only those principles which have special bearing on the present study are indicated here.

both stable (standing patterns) and processual (innovative or disruptive) behavior within these behavior settings must receive careful attention.

Finally, the very act of social research must take the form of symbolic interaction, involving the attempt to reach the level of consensual meanings in the social situation. Central to this interaction is a concept within the setting which enables the researcher to participate in and organize for himself the interaction he is witness to. Thus, both the concept and the methodology act as empirical sensitizers[5] to be employed as observational techniques based upon the premises of symbolic interactionism.

The central concept employed in this study is the *behavior setting* as the unit of observation, and the methodology, that of *participant observation*, both of which are defined below.

THE BEHAVIOR SETTING

A behavior setting may be defined as consisting of three elements: first, the *non-behavioral factors of milieu and time*, which includes space bounded in some fashion that sets it aside from other behavior settings, areas (hereafter referred to as subsettings) located within the general space which are reserved for specialized activities, and time limits which serve as starting and stopping points for behaviors;

---

[5] Blumer, in a discussion of the use of sensitizing concepts, states that "it gives the user a general sense of reference and guidance in approaching empirical instances. Whereas definitive concepts provided prescriptions of what to see, sensitizing concepts merely suggest directions along which to look." (Ibid.:14)

second, *standing behavior patterns* composed of stable, recurring, and taken-for-granted activities of the actors and the interrelated ground rules supporting these activities; and third, the *relationship between the behavioral and the non-behavioral factors* (Gump, 1971:130–134).[6]

The total configuration of the behavior setting is thus defined as consisting of more or less stable elements that actors rely upon and use as the basis of action, as well as the organization of these elements being particularly unique to the setting (Zimmerman and Polner, 1970). In short, the present study will center on the discovery of the practices exhibited by the actors in the chiropractic behavior setting whereby they present to one another the setting as they respond to it situationally.

Focus

While the totality of features and interactional patterns within any behavior setting may be subject to scrutiny, in

[6] It could be construed that for the symbolic interactionist there is an inherent danger in distinguishing between behavioral and nonbehavioral elements: all perceived objects, according to Mead, are, by definition, relative plans of action and as such are inseparable from the temporal and special context within which they are perceived. Although ecological psychologists have recently recommended studying the physical aspects of a setting completely apart from the behavior which takes place within it (see, e.g., Barker, 1968), this seems counter to the traditional interactionist approach. However, a modification of Gump's model as it is used here is defensible on the grounds that it emphasizes the dynamic interplay between heuristically distinguishable elements.

The main modification of Gump's model involves the inclusion of so called rules. Although not posited here as causal elements in an explanatory sense, the actors in the setting, particularly the practitioner, repeatedly referred to and spelled out for me the "rules of the game" which is why they are included here.

the present study the following specific foci are considered essential:

1. *The physical layout of the setting:* front entrance, waiting room, hallway (main traffic flow past the practitioner's office), adjustment area, X-ray room, private office

2. *The rhetoric* or the various forms of impression management designed to convey to the patient and to others the promise and professionalism of chiropractic: written materials (posters, signs, diplomas, pamphlets, professional magazines), oral presentations, office paraphernalia (charts of the nervous system, a skeleton, X-ray equipment) etc.

3. *General expectations within the setting*

4. *Entrance and exit procedures*

5. *Standing behavior patterns*

6. *The ground rules* upon which these relatively stable patterns are based[7]

7. *The form and content of encounters* between actors in the behavior setting (practitioner, patients, supportive others, assistants, other practitioners and professional allies)

8. *Problematic* (disruptive) *behavior*: patients' dissatisfaction, disputes with other practitioners, the restrictive effects of the new state chiropractic laws, business difficulties in general

STUDY DESIGN

Participant Observation

In order to achieve the goals outlined above, an extensive use of the participant observation technique was required.

[7] These are not to be construed as causal in the traditional sense, but are included here primarily because the practitioner insisted that the regularities in his practice were based upon the rules he had learned during the course of his training and his experience in the Clinic.

Initially, I had been a patient participant in the Clinic. Although the primary reason for seeing the practitioner had been one of curiosity, nevertheless I had been suffering from chronic spinal discomfort for which no relief had been afforded by the establishment physicians. During these visits, I became acquainted with the practitioner and his wife, who was his full-time assistant. Moreover, friendly relationships were also established with various regular patients in the Clinic.

After having decided to study the Clinic as a deviant behavior setting, I asked the practitioner if he would employ me as his part-time assistant. Since he had young children and his wife wished to spend more time at home, he readily accepted. At this point in time I shifted from the "natural stance" of the native's position (Natanson, 1962) to that of the interactional analyst (participant observer), while carrying out the duties of assistant. These duties involved general office work, which included the duties of a receptionist and telephone operator.

The chiropractor knew that I was in graduate school and had an interest in "social medicine." He was under the impression, which was largely fostered by himself, that I was considering chiropractic as a profession. For this reason he began to train me in the techniques of chiropractic as well as chiropractic public relations.[8]

As the chiropractor's assistant I was allowed direct contact with all actors in the setting. The position of assistant

[8] This training procedure is not unusual because one of the major concerns of the chiropractor is the recruitment of persons into the profession so that "the world might become aware of this great cause." Application forms for admission to the Palmer College of Chiropractic were on display in the waiting room.

was advantageous because "professional," informal communication became possible with all patients seeing the practitioner. Moreover, "backstage" (Goffman, 1959) data were also easily available and direct quotations were recorded as accurately as possible.

Comparative Data Sources

It has been indicated (Denzin, 1970) that no single method will ever meet the requirements of the interactionist's frame of reference as set forth above. Participant observation, in this case coupled with the sensitizing concept of the behavior setting, must be supplemented with other data sources. Participant observation, as one methodological technique, reveals only certain aspects of empirical reality and, for such reasons, must be supported, ideally, with multiple methods. Denzin has termed this procedure, "triangulation."

Utilizing the triangulation procedure to check the reconstruction of the setting and a patient typology, information from six data sources was compared and contrasted to reveal any discrepancies:

Participant Observation. This main data source, as described above, constitutes the core ethnography.

Unobtrusive Observation.   It might be objected that the continual presence of a participant observer could disrupt the normal flow of interaction in social situations. This was not considered to be a central problem in the Clinic, the role of assistant being an integral part of the performance team. It was felt that unobtrusive observation would serve to cross check statements made by various actors in the setting. The problem of whether an informant actually does what he says he does is an obvious difficulty in any research endeavor.

While carrying out my duties in the Clinic, I had the continuous opportunity to unobtrusively overhear conversations among the patients in the waiting room. Furthermore, I was able to record most of the dialogues which took place between the practitioner and his patients while not being physically present. Finally, most of the telephone conversations of the practitioner were noted without actually participating. As far as could be determined, never was there any attempt to hide any actions or interactions from my observations.[9] It should be added that at no time did I attempt to hide the fact of my observations from either the staff or the patients.

Unstructured, Open-Ended Interviews with the Practitioner. Toward the end of the three-and-one-half-month period of my employment as assistant, I informed the practitioner that I was interested in writing about my experiences in the Clinic in the form of a sociological study. I was careful to point out that he and all the actors in the Clinic would remain anonymous. He was interested in my recorded observations, which were related to him orally, and expressed a desire to help.

---

[9] One of the earliest and most significant works dealing with unobtrusive measures is Webb, et al., *Unobtrusive Measures: Nonreactive Research in the Social Sciences* (1966); see also Denzin, 1970:260–293. As Denzin has indicated, one of the most perceptive applications of the unobtrusive method can be found in Goffman's studies of face-to-face interaction (see esp. 1967).

These interviews lasted on the average of one to two hours a day for a period of two weeks and they took place in his private office. For the most part, he concurred with the observations in this study.

Interviews with the Full-Time Assistant (Wife). Although his wife was present with the practitioner during three of the interviews described above, it was also possible to interview her alone. These interviews, however, were sporadic, usually taking place during those times when the practitioner was occupied.

It should be noted that of all the data sources listed here, the wife contributed the least original information. This was due to the following reasons: she was a full-time assistant only in the early days of the research project and, although she was primarily responsible for my training as assistant in the beginning, she appeared in the Clinic less often after the first two weeks; second, her conception of chiropractic, her husband's professional experience, and her definitions concerning the Clinic and the patients who came to it generally agreed with those of her husband. This of course is also very significant.[10]

Interviews with Patients. As with the interviews which took place with the practitioner and his wife, patient interviews were open-ended, unstructured, and took place during

[10] During the practitioner's chiropractic schooling, his wife became well aware of the type of training he received. She seemed quite knowledgeable concerning chiropractic topics. At the Palmer College of Chiropractic, where the practitioner received his degree, wives of students are encouraged to participate in their husband's practice. Chiropractic schooling is a major social event involving class activities, parties, friendship sessions with wives participating freely. At the chiropractor's graduation, his wife, along with the other wives, received a "GHT" (Getting Hubby Through) degree.

the last days of the study. Patients were informed of my status as a researcher.

A total of thirty-one patients were interviewed and all interviews took place in the waiting room. At times other patients were present, although many were alone when interviewed. Neither the practitioner nor his wife was ever present. The time spent with each patient ranged from ten to forty-five minutes.

A certain amount of selection was necessary to assure the inclusion of patients who had already been typed by the practitioner. The sample was composed of fifteen regular patients, ten problem patients, and six who had been typed as one timers. These patient types will be discussed in detail in Chapter Five which deals specifically with the practitioner's typology.

Interviews with Other Chiropractors. Extensive interviews were obtained from three other chiropractors. They varied in terms of purpose, duration, and the times at which they were conducted during the course of the study.

Before my employment in the Clinic, I visited a chiropractor who practiced in the same building. Although I had been a former patient of the first chiropractor, my visits to his office were prompted primarily by curiosity. After a one-month period—during which I saw him twice weekly—I became familiar with the routine of a chiropractic office.

When the chiropractor later moved to a nearby city, he rented his office to the practitioner who was eventually to employ me. I continued my contact with the first chiropractor and often spoke to him on the telephone. The Clinic's practitioner and I questioned him in detail about various practical aspects of his former practice; for instance, there were questions concerning various patients, the equipment in the office, and rental procedures. Unfortunately, a dispute occurred between the two practitioners, and a follow-up interview at the conclusion of this study became impossible.

Approximately one month before the study was terminated, I visited the only other chiropractor in the town. This practitioner defined himself as a mixer chiropractor. As will be seen, mixer chiropractors strongly disagree with straight chiropractors (and the Clinic's practitioner was a straight chiropractor) about treatment procedure.

Since the two practitioners knew each other casually, each was very interested in the practice of the other. For this reason, it was possible to obtain an extensive one-and-one-half hour interview with the mixer practitioner. The interview was conducted in his office during his regular office hours.

After the study in the Clinic was terminated, I visited, again as a patient, a third chiropractor whose practice closely resembled the practice of the Clinic's practitioner. Since he was also a "straight" chiropractor, he shared a common philosophy. Furthermore, the physical appearance of his clinic, the size of his staff, and the volume of his business were quite similar. His practice was located in a town over a hundred miles from the Clinic in this study; he knew of the Clinic's practitioner only by name.

After being processed as a new patient and receiving a spinal adjustment, I discussed my prior employment in the Clinic, revealed my intentions to write a study based upon those experiences, and asked him to comment on my oral observations. The interview session lasted a little more than one hour. Again, it took place in his office during his regular office hours.

The interviews with the other chiropractors served as sensitizers (Blumer, Ibid.:14). The first straight chiropractor increased my awareness of the practical aspects of running a chiropractic office; the mixer practitioner drew attention to the subtleties of chiropractic philosophy. Both chiropractors served to orient my research within the Clinic and to open new paths of inquiry.

The last chiropractor helped summarize the entire study because he reviewed with me (as did the Clinic's practitioner) my general findings. Also, the patient typology, which had been constructed for me by the practitioner in the Clinic, was examined by the third chiropractor and his observations were noted.

Although it is not the purpose of this study to generalize its findings to all chiropractic clinics, there are reasons for assuming, to a limited extent, trans-situational qualities:

1. The training that most chiropractors receive supplies them with a fairly uniform set of definitions concerning the "business of running a business" and much of their schooling is devoted to this end.
2. Patients coming to the Clinic, who had prior experience in chiropractic clinics elsewhere, encountered little difficulty in adjusting to their new surroundings since they often expressed similar expectations and definitions of the situation.
3. Other chiropractors interviewed responded to the observations contained in this study in a manner which would indicate trans-situational applicability.

PATIENT TYPOLOGY

A typology of patients is presented in Chapter Five (below). The typology was constructed around the characteristics of patients as perceived, organized, and expressed by the practitioner in the Clinic. These types include those persons who came to the Clinic on a regular basis, those who were sporadic in their visits, and those who failed to continue treatment.

The question of patient conversion to this particular deviant form of health care practice hopefully will prove valuable in the study of conversion to other forms of marginal philosophies and/or behavior patterns.[11]

The final chapter constitutes a general summary, review, and a discussion of the implications of the entire study. Suggestions for future research are made.

[11] See John Lofland's *Doomsday Cult: A Study of Conversion, Proselytization and Maintenance of Faith* (1966).

CHAPTER **TWO**

General Chiropractic History, Philosophy, Associations, and the Law

Traditionally, in any sociological work dedicated to the analysis of a specific problem, a review of the historical development of the social phenomena under investigation is given. This material is stated as comprehensively as possible by the researcher and ideally in strictly objective terms.

In the attempt to adhere to the stated principles and objectives of a symbolic interactional analysis as discussed in Chapter One, the following review of chiropractic will be related primarily from the point of view of the central figure in the behavior setting of the Clinic under study: the chiropractor himself. Although this approach may at first seem to have its limitations, it can be justified.

Basically, actors in any social situation use as an orientation for behavior their interpretations of ground rules relative to the perceived biographies of all significant other persons who are relative to that setting. For the Clinic practitioner these significant others included not only those persons with whom he had direct interactional contact in the physical setting (i.e., patients, assistants and, at times, fellow practitioners), but also those persons whom he saw as having contributed to the development of his profession. The leaders of chiropractic espouse a more or less total philosophy of life as well as chiropractic practice, and for this reason they are viewed collectively as a major reference group for most chiropractors.

When recalling the history and philosophy of chiropractic, the Clinic practitioner would frequently quote from the writings of these men. The practitioner's library mainly consisted of philosophical treatises on various chiropractic subjects. This material, termed methodographical source material, was referred to more often than all other writings, including books on physiology or adjustment techniques.

CHIROPRACTIC METHODOGRAPHY:
THE ACTOR AS METHODOLOGIST

Buchler, in his *Concept of Method* (1961), draws an interesting distinction between the terms methodology and methodography. Although both generally refer to the articulation of methods by the professional,[1] methodology—in this case the chiropractic method—consists of the techniques of (1) spinal manipulation for treatment, and (2) impression management (the social front) in the behavior setting. Methodography, on the other hand, refers to the "practi-

[1] Buchler uses as his examples both the scientist and the artist although the chiropractor or any other professional social actor may be discussed in this context.

tioner's discrimination of his methodic process and its aspects" (ibid.: 129). This entails situational and self-evaluation.

Modifying Buchler's schema to fit the chiropractic situation, methodography has a three-fold importance: (1) it enables the practitioner to detect the repeatable elements in his practice, (2) it can stimulate the structure and facilitate interaction between himself and other sympathetic practitioners, and (3) it can serve as supportive data for the practitioner who maintains that only those who have been "dipped" or converted to the philosophy of chiropractic are in a position to engage in abstract study (ibid.:128).

It is from this methodographic activity that the chiropractor seeks to modify, explain, and at times, rationalize his behavior in such a way as to make it coherently presentable to himself and to others. Thus, constructing a chiropractic history from the standpoint of the practitioner necessarily involves the raising of that actor to the traditionally elevated position of the professional researcher (Zimmerman and Polner, 1970).

The following brief account of chiropractic history and philosophy is based primarily upon lengthy discussions with the practitioner and his full-time assistant. Although written in a formal prose style for the reader's convenience, the material itself was gathered informally in an unstructured behavior setting.

The authors, having read widely on chiropractic history[2] and philosophy, became increasingly impressed, throughout

---

[2] Despite McCorkle's statement that there does not exist "a satisfactory history of chiropractic (1961:21)," Turner (1931), Dye (1939), and Wardwell (1951) supply a wealth of background data.

the duration of the study, that the practitioner was extremely well informed and accurate in his descriptions of chiropractic history. This supports Wardwell's (1951:99) observation that a major portion of chiropractic training includes a thorough knowledge of chiropractic history and philosophy.[3]

In the following account, only occasionally was it necessary to elaborate upon the information supplied. Where this is done, it is so noted. With minor exceptions all material, quoted or otherwise, came directly from the practitioner or from written material suggested by him for my edification. All material was discussed with him at length to assure an accurate recording of his interpretations and conceptions of chiropractic.

In the strict sense of the term, the material is subjective as compared to so-called objective reviews of the literature cited above. It is biased in those directions which the practitioner felt most adequately expressed his conception of chiropractic and his position in the field. Most popular reviewers of chiropractic, for example, tend to emphasize its history at the expense of its philosophical beliefs. Yet, the practitioner, in terms of relative significance, saw it otherwise.

The following material is presented in a straightforward fashion without any of the emotional overtones with which

[3] It should be noted that chiropractic education consists mainly of philosophy. In the colleges approved by the Chiropractic Council of Education, a normal four-year curriculum includes courses in human anatomy, physiology, pathology, physical therapy, first aid, spinal analysis, and adjustment techniques. The practitioner, however, repeatedly emphasized, as did the other chiropractors interviewed, that in all courses, even dermatology, a systematic attempt is made to present all material in light of the Principle: the result is a fairly unified body of training held together with Innate Intelligence.

it was sometimes originally related. The chiropractor, when introducing the author to the history and principles of his profession, often became evangelical in his presentation. For the most part, his missionary zeal has been omitted. Specific interpretations and situational applications of this material are to be found in later chapters which deal with the specifics of the behavior setting, for instance, those interactional patterns initiated by the practitioner and his staff which serve to make presentable to all other actors their definition of the situation from which the following information is inextricable.

CHIROPRACTIC HISTORY

The Origins of Chiropractic: The Trinity of Giants

Chiropractors seem to adhere to the "great man" theory of history at least as far as the development of their profession is concerned. Almost invariably, any treatment of the history by sympathetic chroniclers traces the origin of chiropractic to the year 1895. In that year, in Davenport, Iowa, chiropractic was discovered.

Daniel David Palmer: Discoverer of Chiropractic.[4] Of English ancestry, having emigrated from Canada, D. D. Palmer settled in Davenport, Iowa, and although self-educated, worked at several occupations including grocer,

---

[4] One author, however, maintains that Palmer actually rediscovered principles which were known to "the Greeks, Ancient Egyptians, Chinese and Hindus, more than thirty-two centuries ago" (Scofield, 1969). A similar claim is made by Dintenfass (1970).

teacher, and magnetic healer. The latter interest stemmed from the influence of Paul Caster, who espoused magnetic healing based upon the notion of animal magnetism made popular by the Austrian physician Anton Mesmer.

Palmer practiced magnetic healing successfully for ten years before his "Monumental Discovery" of the chiropractic principle. The comment (Wardwell, 1951) that Palmer's account of his first adjustment is "as well known to chiropractors as the biblical story of Eve's creation" is supported by the practitioner's accurate recollection of most of the details in Palmer's account. In Palmer's words:

Harvey Lillard, a janitor in the Ryan block where I had my office, had been so deaf for 17 years that he could not hear the racket of a wagon on the street or the ticking of a watch. I made inquiry as to the cause of his deafness and was informed that when he was exerting himself in a cramped, stooping position, he felt something give way in his back and immediately became deaf. An examination showed a vertebra racked from its normal position. I reasoned that if that vertebra was replaced, the man's hearing should be restored. With this object in view, a half-hour's talk persuaded Mr. Lillard to allow me to replace it. I racked it into position by using the spinous process as a lever and soon the man could hear as before. There was nothing "accidental" about this as it was accomplished with an end in view, and the result expected was obtained. There was nothing "crude" about this adjustment; it was specific, so much so that no Chiropractor has equaled it. [Palmer, 1921:128]

A local Davenport minister and friend of Palmer's, Samual H. Weed, coined the term "chiropractic" from the Greek words *cheir* ("hand") and *praxis* ("practice"). Now named and more or less defined, chiropractic as an organized profession developed slowly in its early years. Practicing for several years in a semisecret manner, Palmer was apparently reluctant to reveal the nature of his technique except to members of his family and close friends.

At the insistence of his son, Bartlett Joshua Palmer—affectionately referred to by the practitioner and most others in his profession as "BJ"—the elder Palmer agreed to expand his practice. In 1897, the Palmer Infirmary and Chiropractic Institute was founded in Davenport.

Although there seems to be some disagreement in the available literature on chiropractic history, the practitioner insisted that Palmer was eventually imprisoned in 1906 for a period of six months for practicing medicine without a license.[5] In that same year "BJ," apparently much more of a businessman than his father, gained controlling interest in the school. Other schools were established in these early years, most of them realizing moderate success.

In 1910, when affiliated with the Pacific College of Chiropractic in Portland, Oregon, Palmer wrote his classic textbook, *The Chiropractor's Adjustor: A Textbook of the Science, Art, and Philosophy of Chiropractic for Students and Practitioners*, which laid out for the first time the truths upon which the profession bases its existence. In spite of this text's early date (or perhaps because of it), the practitioner frequently referred to it as a main source of infor-

[5] Although Dye (1939) does not mention this fact, it is supported by Turner (1931). The practitioner indicated that he had learned it somewhere at college, and took great pride in relating this fact of persecution.

mation and support as he did with other texts of similar vintage.[6]

"BJ" Palmer: Developer of Chiropractic.   Born in 1881 in What Cheer, Iowa, "BJ," like his father, was largely self-educated. Later, he became one of the four students in the Palmer School of Chiropractic (class of 1902). Assisted by his wife, who was the first woman chiropractor, the school prospered.

Often described as one of the most colorful and controversial personalities in chiropractic, "BJ" was also a writer.[7] He aided in the foundation of the first chiropractic association. At the time of his death, he was president of two broadcasting companies, which are both still operating in Iowa as well as president of the Palmer School and the International Chiropractic Association. Extravagant in his ferver, "BJ" combined worldwide travel, extensive lecture tours, and active participation in courtroom battles ("He fought courageously"), bringing widespread attention and excitement to this "revolutionary" form of health care practice.

Willard Carver: Preventive Chiropractic.   Another native Iowan, Carver practiced law for a number of years, specializing in negligence cases. His knowledge of human physiology led him to study chiropractic with D. D. Palmer. Carver is honored for his "distortion-by-Compensation" studies in which he "evaluated the mechanical behavior of the spine and pelvis under all normal and abnormal conditions." He maintained that "not only spinal subluxations (displacements) but also distortions of any and all bodily

[6] The early work was reissued in 1914 by the National Chiropractic Association.

[7] By 1910 he had written five books on chiropractic.

structures create an environment favorable to the development of dis-ease."[8]

Conscientious care and maintenance of the body, which includes correct posture through periodic chiropractic adjustment, can prevent the occurrence of dis-ease (from a section read to me by the practitioner from Dintenfass, 1970:140).[9]

These three individuals, D. D. Palmer, B. J. Palmer, and Willard Carver, are often referred to as the Trinity of Giants in the development of chiropractic. Others of lesser importance are mentioned throughout the literature as having pioneered in diverse ways, for instance, raising educational standards, introducing the X-ray technique, and refining the methods of adjustment.

David D. Palmer, the grandson of the founder of chiropractic, is currently the president of Palmer College. He serves primarily in the capacity of administrator and is not a controversial or outspoken individual. Little reference was made to him by the practitioner as a contemporary spokesman of chiropractic. There are, however, prominant individuals today who serve in the capacity of leaders in the profession. The relationship between the practitioner and these influential persons will be the subject of a later section.

The early history of chiropractic is full of quarrels. There are several accounts of the many disagreements between

[8] "Dis-ease" is a chiropractic play on words; the traditional term "disease" is rejected since it implies the presence of germs.

[9] Although Carver is probably the least discussed person of the three, his contribution is significant and deserves attention since his rationalization of preventive chiropractic serves as the mainstay of the practices of many chiropractors today, including that of the Clinic's practitioner.

"BJ" and his father. These stories were related to me by the practitioner with humorous understanding. He referred to them as "friendly hostilities" and "growing pains." According to him:

What can you expect? This idea [D. D. Palmer's discovery] was completely new . . . revolutionary! Just trying to understand what it was, was hard enough. Words had to be invented. They had to figure out a way to teach it to others. Old "BJ" sure had his work cut out for him. Sure they fought: They fought hard to make it what it is today.

While there were serious disagreements concerning the practical aspect of becoming recognized, there was, and for the most part still is, strong agreement on the central, unifying, philosophical idea of chiropractic: the body's inborn ability to heal itself or its Innate Intelligence.

CHIROPRACTIC PHILOSOPHY

Chiropractic philosophy holds that a Universal Intelligence (the practitioner said, "Call it God if you want to if it makes it easier to understand") created and is maintaining the entire universe. The manifestation of this Intelligence is called Life. The following extracts are from one of the practitioner's college textbooks.[10]

[10] Ralph W. Stephenson's *Chiropractic Textbook*, 1948 edition. The text was given to me during my first days as assistant in the Clinic. Much of the practitioner's teaching was given support by frequent reference to this source. The italic type in the extracts is neither Stephenson's nor mine, but indicates underlining by the practitioner, denoting *special significance for him.*

A specific portion of this intelligence, localized in a definite portion of matter and keeping it actively organized, is called by Chiropractic, Innate Intelligence . . . .

From [the brain] Innate Intelligence sends its controlling forces via the spinal cord through the nerve trunks emitting from the spinal cord and passing through the intervertebral foramina to nerve branches ramifying to all parts of the body. *Perfect adaptation of universal elements for this body, depends upon perfect control by Innate Intelligence.* Perfect adaptation results in health, and imperfect control results in dis-ease . . . .

Owing to the spinal column being the only segmented structure of bone through which the nerve trunks pass, and the possibility of the displacement of its segments, changing the size and shape of the intervertebral foramina, it is possible for subluxations to occur there and offer interference with the transmission of Innate forces indirectly, if not directly. *All dis-ease is thus traceable to impingements of nerve tissue in the spinal column. Chiropractic is a science which consists in having scientific knowledge of this cause of dis-ease and the artistic ability to adjust and correct these displacements of the segments of the spinal column, thereby removing interference with the transmission of Innate forces.* Adjustment does not add any material or forces to the body but allows Innate to restore to normal what it would have had, had there been no interference. . . .

Chiropractic includes the study of all life . . .[11] our studies. . . .

---

11 With regard to the study of all life, I asked the practitioner if this referred to the study of parts of the living body and all the different kinds of illnesses that it was subject to. He replied that I had missed the point. He insisted that the chiropractor is concerned with all of human activity, "not just the condition of our bodies—that's just the beginning—but we have something to say about everything we humans do here on earth."

will be in regard to the human Innate Intelligence . . . . [Stephenson, 1948:1–2]

During our study of the above passages together, the practitioner reminded me that chiropractic is defined as both an art ("the artistic ability to adjust and correct . . . displacements") and a science. He repeatedly emphasized that chiropractic philosophy is a science with a set of terms all its own. Reading to me from Stephenson's text, he warned:

It is quite natural to fail to see the logic of Chiropractic at first. . . . A closer acquaintance with it, however, reveals the absolute truth of its principles . . . . Deductive reasoning is exactly suited to Chiropractic. By assuming a major premise, that there is a Universal Intelligence which governs all matter, every inference drawn from that major premise and subjected to specific scrutiny, stands the test. [Stephenson, ibid.: xx–xxiii][12]

Chiropractic and Religion

One of the topics most frequently discussed by the practitioner was that of the relationship between chiropractic and religion. As will be seen, this is a topic which was often raised by patients.

D. D. Palmer, the founder of chiropractic, extended the religious aspects of that philosophy only as far as that

---

[12] In Appendix B, I have included a list of thirty-three principles of chiropractic philosophy from Stephenson's text. Hopefully these will help summarize what is otherwise a complex and confusing set of ideas, and should also serve to introduce additional terminology.

which he termed "subjective religion," which simply referred to the moral and ethical obligations of the practitioner. "BJ," however, in his missionary zeal, conceived of a chiropractic utopia. In many respects his philosophy may be thought of as a secular religion in that it is all-encompassing in its worldview; it has implications for the totality of social existence. Once again, referring to the textbook, the practitioner read to me:

In accordance with the hopeful idea given by the Universal Cycle,[13] Dr. Palmer's love for the human race and solicitude for the suffering, lead him to hold that chiropractors have a great mission to perform. Not to improve the basic law—this is impossible—but to remove any negative obstructions brought about by perversions of that law, to the further end of a greater and freer expression of what the law of cycles demands in every phase and attribute. If Chiropractic would be allowed to do this, an ideal state of affairs could be brought nearer. This state of affairs which is not impossible for chiropractors to bring about, if they had the chance, would approach the ideal. An ideal state of sociology [sic] is a utopia.

An ideal sociological state would be a country or a world without sickness, insanity, blindness, feeble-minded people, deaf and dumb, backward children, social evils, abnormal reproduction, etc. If chiropractic were given a chance to do its miracles and reasonable time allowed for the results to be brought about, *it could do much;* more than any other human agency has done or can do, in reducing the above named abnormalities to a minimum. This would be a great economic

13 When I asked the practitioner about the meaning of the term Cycle, he explained that it was one of the absolute laws in chiropractic philosophy, and that it refers to all evolutionary changes in the universe.

saving, because there could be fewer public and charitable institutions and penal institutions. [Stephenson, ibid.:336–337][14]

Obviously, this is chiropractic philosophy in its extreme. These views were firmly held, however, by the Clinic's practitioner and were the subject of much methodographic conversation and speculation.

It would be difficult, if not impossible, to document the impact of these thoughts on chiropractic today merely by reviewing the available literature. Yet the practitioner was heavily influenced in this direction, and it must be assumed —he stated so himself—that advocating these extreme views were an integral part of the learning experience at the Palmer School of Chiropractic.

Not all chiropractors, however, adhere to this radical view of the ameliorative powers of chiropractic. Indeed, there exists a division within the profession. Although joined by a common allegiance to a fundamental set of definitive notions concerning the basic nature of chiropractic adjustment, the degree to which the practitioner should make use of other clinical techniques is subject to heated controversy.

CHIROPRACTIC ASSOCIATIONS

During the course of my training, the practitioner was very concerned that I clearly understood the difference between the "true" form of chiropractic and a corruption of it.

[14] Although this account may seem to reflect the extremism and conviction of a dedicated follower, "BJ," in his comments in the opening pages of this text, gives his wholehearted approval and endorsement: "Of *all* the books written and compiled on Chiropractic Philosophy, this is by far the best, not excepting my own" (B. J. Palmer, in Stephenson, 1927:vii).

The International Chiropractic Association

The ICA, one of the two major, national chiropractic associations, is composed of practitioners who adhere to the straight chiropractic belief (as did the Clinic's practitioner) that chiropractors should limit their techniques to spinal adjustment and "let the natural Innate Intelligence of the body take care of itself." Any attempt to incorporate "unnatural" elements into the adjustment process is considered chiropractically improper and in many cases harmful in that they may actually work against or slow down the natural healing powers of the body.

The American Chiropractic Association [15]

The ACA, the second major professional organization, which the practitioner derogatorily referred to as a mixer group, does sanction the use of various techniques, such as heat therapy, enemas (politely referred to as the Colonic Irrigation Technique), specific exercise programs, regulated diet, and electric modalities. The use of these forbidden techniques indicates to the straight chiropractor that there exists the danger that the profession as a whole may eventually sell out to the medical opposition.

The Cleavage.   As Wardwell has observed:

Organized chiropractic is a "shaky structure" due to small membership, the split between straights and mixers, and the lack of any realistic dependence by a practitioner upon the high

---

[15] Previously, the National Chiropractic Association.

regard of his colleagues in order to achieve professional success.
[Ibid.:342]

As a means of increasing my awareness of this cleavage,
the practitioner referred me to the official definitions of
chiropractic held by each organization. The International
Chiropractic Association has defined chiropractic as follows:

The philosophy of chiropractic is based upon the premise that
disease or abnormal function is caused by interference with
nerve transmission and expression, due to pressure, strain, or
tension upon the spinal cord or spinal nerves, as a result of bony
segments of the vertebral column deviating from their normal
juxtaposition.

The practice of chiropractic deals with the analysis of any
interference with normal nerve transmission and expression, the
procedure preparatory to, and complementary to the correction
thereof, by an adjustment of the articulations for the restoration
and maintenance of health; *it includes the normal regimen and
rehabilitation of the patient without the use of drugs or surgery.*
[ICA, 1971:4, 6; emphasis added]

The American Chiropractic Association's definition of chiropractic reads as follows:

Chiropractic practice is the specific adjustment and manipulation of the articulations and adjacent tissues of the body,
particularly of the spinal column, for the correction of nerve
interference and includes the use of recognized diagnostic
methods . . . . Patient care is conducted with due *regard for
environmental, nutritional, and psychotherapeutic factors,* as
well as *first aid, hygiene, sanitation, rehabilitation* and *related*

procedures designed to restore or maintain normal nerve function. [AMA Data Sheet, 1970; emphasis added at the practitioner's suggestion]

The Clinic's practitioner was an avowed disciple of the "true philosophy of straight chiropractic," referring to the mixer in the 'lowest of terms, as "worse than the medicine man" because he "had been taught the truth once, but now he has to be a big shot and play golf at the country club and make a million bucks." According to the practitioner, the medical doctor operates out of ignorance; the mixer from selfish greed. "He [the mixer] knows that people will pay more when you can impress them with gadgets and pills. It's what patients have been taught to expect."

CHIROPRACTIC AND THE LAW

The practitioner was well aware of the legal dangers of mixing chiropractic with other treatment procedures since the foremost occupational hazard confronting the chiropractor is violation of the law.

From time to time both associations issue warnings and various forms of legal advice to their members. Even the ICA, proportedly the standard bearer of straight chiropractic, recognizes the danger of law violation. In its *Confidential Legal Protection Handbook*[16] the ICA cautions against the use or prescription of "devices, substances or measures which constitute therapies in and of themselves." This

---

[16] It was shown to me by the practitioner; no date was given.

clearly is in accordance with the straight approach to chiropractic. Yet, further on, the handbook states:

When chiropractic patients require other therapy, the chiropractor should therefore unhesitatingly refer such cases to those who are qualified to render such service by training and experience.

Clearly a dilemma confronted the practitioner. Although he specifically rejected the germ theory of disease and the accompanying drug combatents advocated by the medical profession, he remained liable, in the eyes of the law, if he failed to recommend the seriously ill patient to an establishment physician.

Chiropractic Licensure

The practitioner took great pride in relating to me the history of licensure in the United States. "As you can see, we've had a long hard battle."

Organized medicine, in the 1880's, succeeded in enacting the Medical Practice Act in all of the states. In almost all instances, these acts were defined in terms of medical and surgical techniques deemed appropriate by established Western medical practitioners. Penalties were established for practicing medicine without a license. From the early years of chiropractic development to the present day, thousands of prosecutions (the practitioner preferred the term "persecutions") have been brought against those in the profession.

In 1913, Kansas was the first state to pass a law regulating the practice of chiropractic. Since that time all states, the most recent being Louisiana,[17] have passed laws regulating chiropractic licensure. (See Appendix A, Chiropractic Act of Louisiana, page 137 below.)[18]

The practitioner was quick to point out to patients the various governmental and nongovernmental programs under which chiropractic is included. They may serve as an indicator of the present growth and status of the profession to date.

1. Federal Government Programs
   a. *Medicaid*. Congress authorized chiropractic services under Medicaid, Title XIX of the Social Security Act. At this time, at least eighteen states provide chiropractic care under Medicaid.
   b. *Federal Civil Service*. All Federal departments and agencies accept statements from doctors of chiropractic for sick leave of any federal employee.
   c. *Income Taxes*. The Federal government permits medical deductions for chiropractic health services under Federal income tax law.
   d. *Immigration Law*. The Federal government recognizes chiropractic colleges as a basis for admitting aliens into the United States with special status as students.
2. State Government Programs
   a. *Licensure*. Chiropractic is an officially recognized health

[17] Not very long ago, about half of Louisiana's chiropractors were taken into court at one time on the charge of practicing medicine without a license. The chiropractors instituted an action against the state board of medical examiners. Eventually brought before the Supreme Court, it was denied a petition for rehearing. The possibilities of licensure in Louisiana appeared slim until the enactment of legislation in 1974.

[18] The Louisiana Act (No. 39) licensing chiropractic—being the most recent in the nation—is included as Appendix A. It is generally indicative of regulations in other states.

profession in all fifty states, the District of Columbia, and in Puerto Rico. Each of these states or jurisdictions has specific laws defining the practice of chiropractic, prescribing requirements for licensure, and authorizing chiropractic services and care.

    b. *Workmen's Compensation.* Claims for chiropractic care are paid by Workmen's Compensation in all fifty states and the District of Columbia.

3. Non-Government Programs

    a. *Commercial Insurance.* Many commercial insurance companies (including most of the private carriers used to administer medicare) include chiropractic in their health and accident policies.

    b. *Health and Welfare Funds of Labor Unions.* Many health and welfare programs of labor unions include chiropractic care (adopted from ICA, 1973:17–18).

The Response to Licensure

While most mixers herald the fact of nationwide licensure (and the mixer interviewed in this study was no exception), the Clinic's practitioner, being a straight chiropractor, discovered this kind of stringent regulation to be a handicap to his professional activity and livelihood. He saw the definite danger of chiropractic becoming "watered down" by those chiropractors who seek to align themselves with the medical opposition for purposes of achieving professionalism. Now that chiropractic is legal and regulated, the practitioner saw the possibility of the profession losing its unique qualities. One day, he angrily observed:

Many of them [the mixers] have lost sight of the Principle. Chiropractic is headed for deep trouble if we don't watch out.

Those goddamned mixers are doing everything they can to make us look like medical doctors.

According to one contemporary chiropractic spokesman in a statement shown me by the practitioner as found in one of the chiropractic magazines located in his waiting room:

Chiropractic reached a peak in the fall of 1922 when the enrollment at Palmer School of Chiropractic was 3600 students. When I attended in 1923, enthusiasm for chiropractic was expressed by all students. They could hardly wait to begin their practice, or to tell the world about the chiropractic principle and its potentialities for getting sick people well. They were proud to be chiropractors and wanted the world to know it. They had explicit faith in the principles of chiropractic and were undaunted by opposition. As a consequence, many went to jail or served time in work houses but they were ready to lay down their lives for the truth as they saw it. [*Sims*, 1972:10].

In the years that followed, however, a definite decrease in interest and enrollment was experienced in chiropractic schools. It became quite obvious that the profession had lost something and the problem remained as to what could be done to recapture the spirit and enthusiasm which once had characterized it.

NEW LIFE FOR CHIROPRACTIC: DR. SID WILLIAMS AND DYNAMIC ESSENTIAL

Today, one of the acknowledged leaders of those chiropractors who advocate the straight or "natural" approach to chiropractic philosophy and practice is Sid E. Williams

(B.S., D.C.), a friend and advisor to the Clinic's practitioner.

According to the practitioner, and to several chiropractic magazine articles given to me by him, Dr. Sid—as he is known in the profession—was a former football star. Having received a serious injury, he was so successfully cured of it through chiropractic that he entered the profession. He now leads a vanguard movement which espouses the notion of Dynamic Essential with which he proports to express and revitalize the Great Principle discovered by the elder Palmer. His stated goal is to instill in chiropractors the "dedication . . . of D. D. Palmer, his son B. J., and grandson David Palmer." He urges them to "reach for the stars and the 'space ship of dynamic motivation' will take you to unprecedented heights." (1973:8). Williams further promises a "redirected life that can lead . . . to day-by-day success, happiness, and prosperity like you've dreamed possible" [sic] (1973:24).

Realizing the necessity of a dynamic public relations program, his professed intention is to "carry the message" to the people. As founder and president of the "non-profit" organization, The Life Foundation, Williams publishes the periodical, *Health for Life*, which is mailed by chiropractors to potential patients[19] and was found on the waiting room tables of all three chiropractors interviewed in this study.

An avid organizer, Williams promotes several "D. E. Jubilees" and "Homecomings" in major cities throughout the year. Judging from the promotional descriptions of these occasions which appear in chiropractic trade maga-

---

[19] This tactic neatly avoids many of the advertising restrictions imposed by most states.

zines and from the practitioner's eye-witness testimony, these meetings are characterized by a revivalistic spirit. According to the practitioner, "when we [wives, children, and assistants are encouraged to attend] come back from seeing these great people at one of these meetings, I'm up for a month. He's the guiding spirit in chiropractic today."

In addition to being a highly successful businessman, Dr. Sid serves as troubleshooter for chiropractors around the country, giving free advice on the running of a practice and offering personal encouragement and spiritual support.

The Clinic's practitioner drew heavily upon the encouragement and words of advice from this supportive other person in such a way that when personal and professional difficulties arose for him, sympathetic understanding and, at times, ameliorative actions were available. His relationship with Dr. Sid as a supportive other will receive attention in a later section dealing with backstage behavior.

This chapter has dealt with a general overview of the history, philosophy, and current development of chiropractic primarily as it was perceived by the practitioner in the Clinic. Accuracy is not the main concern here, although all information received from the practitioner was checked against fairly objective literature for errors or distortions. But, of central importance is the manner in which the practitioner selectively perceived the information made available to him through his training and experience and how he passed this information on to me. By such an accumulation of data, the practitioner, as researcher, was enabled to methodographically assess, rationalize, and modify his methodology in the behavior setting. Indeed, the behavior setting itself, as defined in Chapter One, is determined, for the most part, by the practitioner's methodographic activity both prior to and during his practice.

The following chapter is devoted to a descriptive analysis of the spacial and temporal properties of the Clinic as a behavior setting.

CHAPTER **THREE**

The Behavior Setting

A behavior setting has been defined above as consisting of: (1) nonbehavioral elements of milieu and time which includes bounded space, objects, areas (subsettings), and time limits; (2) standing behavior patterns; and (3) the relationship between the behavioral and nonbehavioral factors.[1] Any behavior setting consists of these more or less stable elements, which actors use as the basis of their actions. Moreover, these elements are unique to each setting.

In order to ultimately discover those practices exhibited by actors in the Clinic whereby they present to themselves and to one another the setting as they respond to it situationally, each of the above features must be examined in detail. This is the purpose of the present chapter.

An effort has been made to show how the practitioner and his staff utilize presentational devices (stage props) within the setting to give to his patients, and especially his

[1] It should be reemphasized that this distinction is a heuristic one, similar, say, to the distinction normally made between status and role, and is used solely for purposes of analytical description.

new patients, a feeling of confidence in what has been demonstrated to be a deviant setting (see p. 4, above).[2]

EXTERIOR CHARACTERISTICS

The chiropractic office was located in the central part of a small town in a Southern state. Directly across from the Clinic was the city police department. The building immediately adjacent to the Clinic was the largest and most respectable church in town. The Clinic itself was located in a two-story, renovated structure which housed a bank, and on the other side, a flower shop.

The residents of this mixed commercial/residential neighborhood were established, white, and middle class; many were retired. The town population as a whole, however, was heterogeneous in that both black and white neighborhoods were interspersed.

A large white sign, prominant against the dark wood exterior of the building, advertised the Clinic's presence. A heavy glass door, upon which were posted office hours,

[2] As one critic has observed (Douglas, 1970:15–16), a possible weakness in Ball's study of an abortionist's attempt to accomplish this same end—relieving patient anxiety—is that it is dangerous to infer intentionality or meaning to the behavior of actors (see Ball, 1967). Like Roebuck and Frese (forthcoming) I am not concerned with actors' consciousness but with how directly observable impressions are created and sustained. Whereas in their study of an after-hours club, they mention that the staff "appear to be . . . only dimly 'conscious'" of impression management, the practitioner in the present study was quite conscious of this activity. Much backstage conversation testifies to this fact and, as such, is empirically admissible data.

marked the only entrance. Patients entered directly from the sidewalk, ascending two concrete steps.

THE WAITING ROOM

The waiting room (approximately 10x15 feet) was directly visible from the street. Uncarpeted, it was furnished by a central table surrounded by several chairs placed against the walls. Directly opposite the entrance was a wall behind which was located the private office of the practitioner. A shoulder-level sign-in counter was located in the center of this wall, affording the chiropractor and his assistants a panoramic view of the waiting room and the sidewalk outside. Usually an FM radio, tuned to relaxing music, conveyed the impression of serious quietude.

The waiting-room walls, made of inexpensive, unpretentious wood paneling, were heavily decorated with pictures, signs, and posters—all of which communicate the chiropractic message with an air of professionalism. The largest and most impressive of these was entitled "Chiropractic Defined."[3] Also included as part of the wall decorations was a prominant picture of the practitioner's graduating class, which closely resembles that of any large establishment university.

While all of the above are intended to impress upon the patient an atmosphere of competent professionalism, there were also found on the walls a number of handwritten signs

[3] See page 38 above, ICA definition.

expressing a form of homespun philosophy or message for everyday living and/or health care: "An ounce of prevention is worth a pound of cure"; "Many automobiles get better care than most human bodies"; "A stitch in time not only saves nine, but often a human life"; "The graveyards are filled with those who neglected regular care of their health." Although these messages seemed unprofessional, it will later be seen that they played an important part in conveying the message of chiropractic philosophy. As the practitioner expressed it:

It affects everything you do, say, feel and think. Chiropractic is an art. . . . You must reexamine your whole life and the way you live it. These little signs get people to thinking.

The signs, which were changed frequently, were the topic of conversations between the staff and patients and were used expressly for that purpose. "It's a natural. Everybody is interested in living and life. When I talk about the meaning of life and death, people got to listen." These handwritten messages were found throughout the Clinic, and they were placed purposefully in strategic locations.

Admission to the Clinic

Admission was similar to the routines found in many establishment medical settings: the prospective patient went to the admissions window, was greeted by the chiropractic assistant,[4] and signed in. No attempt to secure any informa-

---

[4] It should be noted that the assistant, like the practitioner himself, wears no special clothing other than ordinary street apparel. The practitioner, in trying to convey the image of chiropractic as "simple and

tion other than name and address was made at this time. The patient was always asked to sit down and make himself comfortable. Attention was directed to the magazines and pamphlets, which had been placed on the central table and on several chairs.[5] All of the reading materials pertained directly to the nature and purpose of chiropractic and/or natural health care. Magazines (*Today's Chiropractic, Health, Prevention*), booklets (*Chiropractic Could Save Your Life*), newspapers (*Spinal Column*), and pamphlets ("Chiropractic: An Explanation"; "Why Chiropractic?") engaged the patient's attention.[6]

During the waiting period in which the practitioner may or may not have been busy ("The patient expects to wait . . ."), the assistant attempted to engage the patient in casual conversation. Topics such as the weather were discussed. If the patient asked a question concerning chiropractic or related topics, the subject was actively pursued. The assistant saw this as an opportunity to "dip," or convert, the patient into the general philosophy and orientation of chiropractic. The dipping procedure was an integral part of the overall rhetoric and was pursued whenever the opportunity afforded itself. Although the assistant attempted to stimulate interest and curiosity, a line was drawn whenever specific questions concerning the philosophy or adjust-

---

natural," felt that to wear a white jacket of the establishment physician was inconsistent to this end. However, it should be added that some chiropractors, especially mixers, choose to wear white jackets in order to promote their professional image.

[5] Many chiropractors often leave a copy of the Bible, opened to an appropriate passage, in a conspicuous place.

[6] As Goffman has noted, newspapers and other reading material in public places serve to offer to actors a "minimal involvement" whenever the individual "feels he ought to have an involvement but does not" (1963:51–52).

ment technique arose. One patient was heard to ask the assistant:

If what it says here [referring to an article in one of the chiropractic magazines] is true, then I should be feeling better in a couple of weeks. Right?

The assistant replied:

That's a good question. A lot of people ask the same thing. There's really no easy answer, but the Doctor is a lot better at explaining it than I am. Be sure to ask him when you go in.

Often the assistant would brief the practitioner concerning the nature of the question or concern, thus allowing for preparation of an answer.

Many times regular patients were allowed to enter immediately into the adjustment area without going through the process of signing in. For these patients the atmosphere was much less formal, and they were made to feel at home by being welcomed on a first-name basis. In numerous instances the assistants and the practitioner were addressed informally. This was encouraged in patients defined as having been thoroughly dipped into the philosophy of chiropractic.

Immediate entry was also given to those patients, either new or regular, who state any need to see the practitioner. This was done sometimes at the expense of making other patients extend their wait. When asked about the fairness of this practice, the practitioner replied:

Oh come on! I'm running a business here. I'm not going to let five bucks walk out the door. I've got kids to feed. Most people don't know the difference anyway. They think he's got an appointment. If I don't get my hands on him the first time, I'm sure as hell not going to get him again.

The decor of the waiting-room entrance presented to the patient what appeared to be a respectable and, for the most part, conventional front.[7] Many prospective patients, upon entering the Clinic for the first time, were apprehensive and expressed an inadequate definition of the situation. By giving the patient time to become adjusted to the surroundings and some indication as to the ground rules, the aura of mystery associated with chiropractic was to some extent alleviated. As one regular patient confided to a new patient:

I didn't know what to expect. I'd heard a lot of goofy things and I didn't even want to come the first time, but my boss told me it would get me back to work fast if I did, so I came. After you find out what it's all about is when it begins to do you some good. They're pretty good people here.

Various attempts were made by the Clinic's personnel to relate to the patients by structuring personal encounters. Often, when a known patient was observed approaching the front door, his card was quickly pulled from the file and all pertinent personal information was reviewed. Questions concerning the well-being of the patient's family, his state of health, or any other personal matter served to draw the individual into the immediate behavior setting. Patients,

[7] Like Ball (1967) and Roebuck and Frese (forthcoming), I have extended Goffman's definition of "front," which included setting, appearance, and manner as a framework for the analysis of self presentation to the overall establishment and the actors within it (Goffman, 1959:22–30).

particularly regulars, responded favorably to this tactic. Some patients were observed reciprocating this personal attention by bringing gifts of flowers, cookies, etc., to the staff.

Not all patients responded positively to this "just-plain-folks" treatment, however. One patient was heard commenting to a friend outside the Clinic, "I come in here 'cause I got bad trouble in my back, and she [the assistant] wants to talk about my family. Hell, that's none of her business!" These varying patient responses were important for the practitioner in that they served as the basis for his classification of patients into one of a series of types and consequently structured both the form and the content of future interaction with them.

THE ADJUSTMENT AREA SUBSETTING

After a waiting period, which was situationally judged appropriate, the patient was told, "The doctor will see you now. Will you come through the door on your right?" The door was opened by the assistant and the patient was led down a narrow hallway, past the practitioner's private office, toward the adjustment area, which constituted the primary behavior subsetting in the total configuration of the Clinic.

The hallway, through which the patient passed, was unadorned except for a large bulletin board on the right directly across from the entryway to the private office. This board posted information of a seemingly more transitory nature than other forms of written rhetoric found elsewhere in the Clinic. They included newspaper clippings and articles (all undated) which denounced various kinds of drugs (e.g., aspirin, vaccines, etc.). Other similar newsworthy items relative to chiropractic were seen, conveying the impression of an immediate awareness and concern for current health care issues. Most of these clippings had been reproduced, thus concealing the fact that some were as much as thirty years old. Also affixed to the board were photographs of the practitioner, garbed in the traditional graduation gown and holding his diploma, as well as several pictures of his children. Three of the handwritten messages were also interspersed.

If the patient had been accompanied to the Clinic by one or more supportive others, the assistant or the practitioner would encourage, and in many cases recommend, that these persons accompany the patient to the adjustment area. This was an important procedure and will be discussed at some length in a following chapter.

The Scene

The adjustment area was the largest room in the Clinic (15x25 feet) and served as the center of all patient-oriented interaction. Descending one step from the end of the hallway, the room was seen to be fully enclosed, windowless, and without outside exit. Wall-to-wall carpeting and soft fluorescent lights set into soundproof ceiling lent an atmosphere of quiet seclusion and privacy. The walls, like those of the waiting room, were of dark, conservative paneling. A door on the left opened upon a small bathroom, and on the right another door, left ajar (see footnote 2, p. 48), exposed an impressive array of X-ray equipment.

Central to the adjustment area itself, however, was the adjustment table, which was located in "upper stage right" (on the left as one enters the room from the hall). Technically known as the Zenith-Thompson Pneumatic Terminal-Point Chiropractic Adjustment Table, it presented a formidable appearance to the new patient. Standing upright, it was seen to be constructed of four vinyl-covered sections: (1) the FM (forward motion) head piece, composed of two spaced sections covered with a wide strip of replaceable tissue paper for the patient's face; (2) the dorsal-lumbar section, also constructed of two parallel pieces; (3) the pelvic section, which supported the pelvis and the legs; and (4) a small ankle support section. Each section could be adjusted to conform to the height and proportions of each individual patient. Additionally, the pelvic section was equipped with a mechanical device triggered with a remote control foot pedal, which allowed this section to suddenly drop a short distance and return to its original position automatically. While the device was in an upright position, the patient stepped upon a small platform resting on the floor. The entire table was then mechanically lowered to the floor with an electrical humming sound. The underside of the table, now beneath the upholstered cushions, revealed the impressively complex mechanics of the machine: chrome-plated gears, the motor, as well as various tubes and wires. Thus, an advertisement directed to perspective buyers read: "No table today has so many advantages for doctor and patient."

The table was placed approximately 3 feet from the wall,

thus allowing the practitioner to move freely around the prone patient. When the adjustment was completed the table was returned to an upright position, permitting the patient to easily step backward and away.

Directly opposite the adjustment table, close to the facing wall, several straight-backed chairs surrounded a small card table upon which was placed a note pad, pens, pencils, blank patient information cards, blood pressure gauge, and an assortment of brochures and pamphlets.

Attached to the rear wall were two large charts—one depicting the nervous system, and the other a rear view of the skeletal structure of the human body. Both focused upon the spinal column. The charts had been commercially printed with details of precise anatomical terms. Also, in the center of the same wall, hung a replica of the human skeleton, minus appendages. The skeleton faced the wall, exposing the spine. Pieces of thin multicolored cord had been interwoven between the vertebra, demonstrating the major and minor nerves as they led to various parts of the body.

In addition to these prominent and professionally appearing demonstration devices, affixed to the walls of the adjustment area were more handwritten signs. The content of these messages, however, varied somewhat from those found in the waiting room and elsewhere in the Clinic. In the words of the practitioner, they were designed to

. . . make people think about chiropractic and what it's all about. I mean, when you get people to really wonder about what makes your heart beat ("WHAT MAKES YOUR HEART KEEP BEATING? THINK ABOUT IT!"), they're getting dipped, whether they know it or not. DE [Dynamic Essential]

is what this thing is all about. You've got to have faith in it. You can't come right out and tell them, they'll laugh at you.

A frequently used aid in promoting and selling the idea of the Life Force, which was so central to the orientation and philosophy of the ICA chiropractor, was a large hand-written poster that had been placed adjacent to the table and chairs. It read:

RESISTANCE CHART

Complete Health	100%	LIFE
Not Feeling Well	75%	LIFE
Sick	50%	LIFE
Very Sick	25%	LIFE
Dead	0%	LIFE

How Is Your Resistance?

For those patients who had complained of a specific ailment or discomfort, a pamphlet rack, constructed of perforated board and wire hangers, was used to dispense information. These small, one-page, "fact sheets" were free, and the patients could take as many as they wished for their own use or to "give to friends or relatives who may need some good, sound, practical advice." The rack itself hung within easy reach of the practitioner while seated with patients around the table.

Completing the wall rhetoric in the adjustment area was a Chiropractic Prayer. It had been commercially reproduced as the standard prayer for all ICA chiropractors, and it was endorsed by that organization. Essentially it was an appeal to a higher power, without reference to any specific religious denomination, including Christianity, for help in the effective use of the hands in order to ameliorate "the pain in this troubled world." This higher power, which was never explicitly defined, was referred to variously by the practitioner as Innate Intelligence, the Wisdom of the Body, Dynamic Essential, or Life Force.

Some patients openly discussed this topic and expressed their understanding of it in purely objective, biological terms: nerve energy did not seem to pose much of a problem to the practical patient. Others, however, responded quite differently. An elderly female patient, who had been seeing the practitioner for some months on a regular basis, confided to the researcher:

I surely do like that man. I do believe what he says. He's got a lot of schooling . . . [but] he talks to me like a friend. I ain't never had a real doctor talk to me about the Spirit like he does.

The adjustment area subsetting was characterized by a façade of respectable professionalism carefully combined with a "down to earth" hominess. The practitioner, in a purposeful way, used the setting and its components in a highly efficient presentation of a non-threatening, yet professionally powerful, self-image.

THE X-RAY SUBSETTING

Patients entering the X-ray room with the practitioner observed it to be fairly small (8 x 10 feet) and filled with standard, yet complex equipment: the X-ray machine itself;

a lead backdrop shield; racks of exposed negatives, many of which were hanging on the walls and always one on the lighted viewer; several wall charts covered with complicated mathematical figures, diagrams, and procedural instructions. The room was designed for efficiency and was the only one in the Clinic devoid of extraneous trappings or decorations. The absence of carpet contributed to the tone of clinical austerity. The only adornment was the wooden wall paneling found in all other rooms.

The technique utilized by the chiropractor was referred to as spinography or spinal radiography. The practitioner took pictures according to standard procedure, producing a classical spinography of the entire spinal column, and smaller pictures, usually a detail of the neck and pelvic areas from both back and side views.

The X-ray room was the only subsetting area in use denied access to the author, for reasons of protection. It can be assumed, however, that little interaction took place during this period of isolation for the following reasons: (1) the practitioner was indeed concerned with producing pictures of clarity and precision and must therefore be conscientious of technique; (2) relatively little time was spent in the area other than the time normally required for taking the pictures; and, (3) the practitioner stated that the setting was not truly conducive to conversation with the patient, the latter usually was asked to return to the adjustment area and wait while last minute details of the X-ray procedure were completed.

It should not be concluded that the time spent in the X-ray setting was unimportant from a behavioral point of view. The procedure and the photographs served to promote interest, confidence, and commitment in the patient. When the pictures were placed in the patient's file, it produced a sense of belonging and self-identification with the Clinic and with chiropractic in general.[8]

The practitioner, returning to the adjustment room and the waiting patient, seated himself at the interview table to review the patient's problem. Literature was dispensed along with advice concerning "the home care of the spine."[9]

THE HALLWAY SUBSETTING AS
TERMINATION POINT

In most cases the practitioner made the decision of when the adjustment area interview was concluded, unless the patient took it upon himself to leave. Normally the patient followed the practitioner back through the hall, at the end of which was the door to his private office on the right. Opening the door as they entered, the practitioner seated himself at his desk next to the file cabinet, leaving the patient standing in the doorway. Posted conspicuously on the door was a neatly lettered poster designating fees:

[8] It is not uncommon for chiropractors, when learning that a patient is going out of town for several days or weeks, to give him his X-rays and a list of chiropractors (in this case, ICA members) located en route. This practice serves two functions: reciprocal agreement between chiropractors assures a higher volume of business for each, and an emphasis on the importance of returning the pictures assures the return of the patient also.

[9] Such advice may include rest periods to allow the body to respond "naturally" to the adjustment, proper sleeping positions, and possibly some appropriate series of exercises.

First Visit	$ 5.00
X-ray	$10.00
Advanced Payment	$40.00
10 Visits (Save $10.00! ! !)	
Second Member of Family	$4.00
Additional Family Members	$1.00

Never any more than $10.00 for the entire family.

At this point the practitioner briefly reviewed the patient's case and recommended an appropriate time for the next appointment. This appointment was based on the "physical needs" of the patient. After this had been established, the fee was discussed, pointing out the advantages of the prepay plan. Patients were usually encouraged to tell family members of the beneficial treatment they had received with the hope they would bring others with them at the next visit. When the matters of appointment and fees had been settled, the conversation terminated on a friendly and encouraging note.

As will be seen in the following chapter, hallway interaction is of major concern when attempting to understand other aspects of the behavior setting. The patient was free to raise questions, and often was encouraged to do so, concerning any aspect of chiropractic. Often the bulletin board —easily seen by the patient—was made the focus of attention. The practitioner could direct the patient's attention to an article or item of interest which had been posted there specifically for this purpose. Whereas in the waiting room, the adjustment area, or the X-ray area the form and content of the interaction had been guided, for the most part, by the practitioner or an assistant, the "burden of proof" in the hallway setting was now purposefully accorded the patient. Depending upon the practitioner's reading of the patient's definition of the situation, including the practitioner's projection of self-image, he typed the patient in terms of future behavioral expectations.

BACKSTAGE SUBSETTING

The practitioner's private office, while open to view for the patient during the course of his visit, was nonetheless actually closed to him in that he was denied access to much of the interaction which took place there at other times. The wood-paneled room itself (12x15 feet) was sparsely furnished, the most prominent feature was the wall-to-wall bookshelf directly facing the hall entry. The practitioner's desk and an upright file cabinet were directly opposite the sign-in window. The telephone was within easy reach of the desk. Three straight-backed chairs completed the floor furnishings. The walls displayed a variety of items, the most prominent of these being the practitioner's framed diplomas from the Palmer College of Chiropractic. They were arranged in a way as to be easily seen from the waiting room through the sign-in window. They included the diploma of Doctor of Chiropractic, a Certificate of Proficiency—X-ray, and a Certificate of Merit.[10] Also given a position of central

[10] The significance of the latter is somewhat questionable in that the practitioner admitted to me that it was awarded as the consequence of "grading some exam papers one semester for an instructor at the college. Everyone gets it."

prominence was a sign printed in boldface script and "signed" by Thomas Edison:

The doctor of the future will give no medicine but will interest his patients in the care of the human frame and in the cause and prevention of dis-ease.[11]

Several of the handwritten signs were also evident: "Children Learn What They Live"; "It Takes 65 Muscles To Frown and Only 13 To Make a Smile—Why Not Smile?"; "It Is Easier To Stay Well than To Get Well." A lighted candle placed upon the sign-in shelf ("A candle loses nothing by lighting another candle. We're here to help you.") added to the decor.

The background music from the radio assured a certain degree of privacy in this backstage area when there were patients in the waiting room, as did the level of the sign-in window which was located above eye level when patients were seated. It was possible to converse in low tones in the office and be assured of not being overheard.

The professional performance team,[12] consisting of the practitioner and his assistants, utilized this backstage area as their central meeting place. During those periods when there were not any patients in the Clinic, the practitioner and his staff would spend their free time in this subsetting.

Occasionally during these interim periods the practitioner would suggest to his staff members moving to the adjustment area for conversation and/or adjustments. The practitioner, as a "true believer" in chiropractic, encouraged

[11] Available from Palmer College, $3.50, without frame.
[12] Defined by Goffman (1959) as "any set of individuals who cooperate in the staging of a single routine."

those backstage others—assistants, family, friends and professional allies—to undergo adjustment routinely.[13]

This chapter has focused upon the physical and temporal essentials of the total configuration of the behavior setting of the Clinic. Furthermore, standing patterns of behavior for the new patient have been outlined. In the following chapter both onstage and backstage interaction as it occurs against this dramaturgical backdrop will be discussed.

---

[13] The author, during the course of his employment, underwent an average of five adjustments a week, despite the fact that the average patient is told for what are apparently purely economic reasons that adjustments are not normally needed on a daily basis.

CHAPTER **FOUR**

Subsetting Interaction

The previous chapter was primarily concerned with the delineation of nonbehavioral features (time and space characteristics) and standing patterns of behavior in the Clinic. This section focuses upon the interplay between the two.

In a traditional health care setting, behavior is less problematical, conscious impression management is minimal, and the social atmosphere is not strained. The chiropractor, on the other hand, is repeatedly confronted with a variety of patients who experience great difficulty in defining the situation. As will be later demonstrated, not all patients respond to the elements in the setting in the same way.

When patients were exposed to the physical–temporal elements and the contrived plans of action in the Clinic, their responses generated interactional problems for the practitioner, who in turn had to reciprocate in a fashion appropriate to the situation.

Continuing in the manner established in the last chapter, this section will accompany the reader through the Clinic, following standing patterns of behavior from one subsetting to another. Typical interaction between the practitioner and his staff and various types of patients will be presented. The actual typing of these patients by the practitioner is the subject of the following chapter.

THE WAITING ROOM: SITUATIONAL INTERACTION

The prospective patients entering the Clinic for the first time were generally unprepared for what awaited them.[1] Except for what they had possibly been told by more experienced patients, they had to rely upon a general set of expectations derived from past experiences in the offices of medical doctors. As one patient explained:

I guess I knew there would be a waiting room and a nurse, but I didn't know what to expect. He calls himself a doctor and I figure his office would look like . . . you know, a doctor's office.

The conservative appearance of the waiting room tended to relieve some of the anxiety expressed by new patients. The wall rhetoric[2] served to neutralize the deviant reputation of the chiropractic Clinic. According to an older man who had come to the Clinic accompanied by his wife:

When we first came in and saw the magazines and the furniture, I kinda knew where I was . . . . When the secretary[3] said "hi"

[1] A review of the content of waiting room interaction indicates that there does not exist for the general public a clear set of definitions concerning what "a chiropractic clinic looks like." Due to the deviant status of chiropractic health care practice, persons are reluctant, it seems, to make public their experiences.

[2] See Ball's comments on the rhetoric of legitimization (1967).

[3] An indication of the general lack of an adequate definition of the situation is indicated by the confusion in role terminology. The chiropractic assistant has been addressed by the new patient variously as "secretary," "nurse," "girl," "helper," "sign-in girl," etc.

and was real nice I didn't worry too much any more. When we came up to the door we still weren't real sure if we were going to come in. . . .

Meaningful human interaction implies intentionality relative to the perceived intentions of others. When there is no basis available for the perception of these intentions (definition of the situation), of course no focused interaction is possible.

Interaction patterns in the waiting room depended primarily upon whether or not the actors involved were experienced or inexperienced patients. Although the waiting room was the most open region in the total configuration (patients, supportive others, assistants, the janitor, the mailman and others were continually entering and leaving the area), conversation was usually held to a minimum in spite of no formal conversational restrictions.

Unfocused Interaction

Waiting room interaction was generally unfocused in that it was limited to simple acknowledgements of the other's copresence. The chiropractic magazines, pamphlets, and brochures which had been made available were almost invariably taken up by the new patient, allowing for minimal involvement in the setting and precluding the uncertainty of a main involvement with others.[4]

Typically the waiting room was occupied by persons unknown to each other, and they constituted an unfocused

[4] These so-called emergency supplies, which are placed in public places, are seen by Goffman as assisting in the prevention of self-exposure and "over-presence" (1963:51–52).

gathering. There was, for the most part, an absence of formal group organization in the sense of a mutually agreed upon set of rights and obligations. The one exception to this was the matter of turn-taking. As indicated above (p. 51) patients entering the Clinic sign-in and thus ordered themselves in terms of behavioral priorities. The signing-in procedure served as a claiming mechanism for the patients and supplied them with a time orientation within the setting. Their relationship with the others was now clarified, and they had some basis for determining a situational course of action for themselves and others present.

The situational definitions (or lack of them) unique to the chiropractic setting—as distinct from those characteristic within the more familiar medical doctor's office—became obvious when the behavior of persons known to each other is examined. Occasionally a prospective patient, when entering the Clinic for the first time, would encounter a friend, neighbor, or someone familiar. In an establishment medical setting a surprise encounter might naturally develop into a prolonged discussion of each individual's illness, treatment, doctor-patient relationship, and other topics of a more or less personal nature. Often this conversation would be carried out within the hearing distance of others.

Interactional encounters between chiropractically inexperienced acquainteds, however, differed markedly. The following conversation (which uses fictional initials or first names in all cases) is illustrative of the conversational restraint observed even among those persons intimately acquainted *outside* the Clinic's setting.[5] Mrs. Z. had been

---

[5] It was learned since this observation was recorded that the participants lived in the same neighborhood, attended the same church, and on several occasions had visited each other in their homes.

seated quietly alone in the waiting room for approximately twenty minutes when Mrs. X. entered. Both had had no previous experience with chiropractic care either in the Clinic or elsewhere.

Mrs. X. [after quickly surveying the waiting room and seeing Mrs. Z.]: Uh . . . well, hi. Good morning.

Mrs. Z.: It's pretty . . . it's too early for me [short laugh] . . . can't wake up. How 'bout you? [Although Mrs. Z had started to continue some line of conversation, Mrs. X. quickly moved to the sign-in window and was greeted by the assistant and was asked to sign in. Mrs. Z. returned to her magazine. Although a seat was available immediately adjacent to the one occupied by Mrs. Z., Mrs. X. selected one several chairs away and picked up some reading material from the central table.]

Mrs. Z.: I *thought* I saw you drive by a few minutes ago but I wasn't sure.

Mrs. X.: Yeah, same old car . . . finding a parking space gets harder all the time. How's [husband] Henry? I heard he was sick.

Mrs. Z.: Oh, he's fine. Working everyday.

Mrs. X.: Well that's fine. [Both return to their reading.]

Mrs. Z. [after several minutes]: Been here long?

Mrs. X.: Not too long.

Again the conversation was terminated and was not picked up again. Mrs. Z., being told "the Doctor will see you now," walked directly past her friend and entered the hall door with no noticeable eye contract or other form of copresence acknowledgement with Mrs. X. When she left, a short but friendly farewell served to terminate the encounter.

At no time during this or similar encounters between in-experienced acquainted persons did the subjects of specific ailments, chiropractic experience, or similar topics become the focus of attention of these persons.

The Necessity of Focused Interaction

The practitioner was well aware of the situational difficulties faced by the new patient. Much of the backstage conversation[6] between practitioner and staff involved discussions of the importance of the assistant-patient relationship. We were urged to "get involved with the patient." The general office duties of the assistant were incidental to the primary task of interaction stimulation.

That dramaturgical discipline and loyalty are main concerns for the performance team in the Clinic was evidenced by the training procedure I experienced when first beginning the job of assistant. After having been "immersed" in the chiropractic philosophy and familiarized with the techniques employed, I was carefully supervised during the first days of my apprenticeship. The trained assistant was left in charge of my patient-relationship training whenever the practitioner was occupied elsewhere. It was repeatedly emphasized that

. . . these people don't know what's going on. We've got to make them feel at home and let them know that there's nothing to be scared of. Be friendly. Talk to them and get them to relax.

The practitioner was indeed aware of the role-playing nature of the assistant's performance in the waiting room:

[6] Discussed on p. 94 below.

Look. It's going to take you a long time to learn what this is all about . . . but you've got to let that patient know that he's in good hands. You don't have to talk chiropractic. In fact you might even confuse them. Just make them think that this place is the nicest place on earth.

Focused Encounters

The chiropractic assistant occupies what Goffman (1963: 128–31) has termed an "opening position" in that he has the license to approach those persons in the waiting room with whom he is unacquainted. In a sense he is a host whose recognized duties necessarily involve direct contact with patients. The assistant not only has the right to initiate encounters but is obligated to initiate face engagements of welcome during the sign-up procedure with all entering the Clinic. The structured interaction which follows, however, is different in two respects from that which is normally observed in the office setting of the medical doctor.

First, the receptionist–patient relationship in the establishment doctor's office is normally an end in itself, initiated to secure specific information concerning the patient's medical background. This was not the practice in the Clinic. For reasons that will become clear later, the assistant intentionally avoided eliciting information concerning the patient's ailments.

A second distinction, closely related to the first, pertains to the directional flow of interaction. Whereas in the medical setting, the assistant opens a channel of communication through which the patient is expected to respond, in the Clinic the assistant initiated and sustained the flow of communication by supplying a set of definitions concerning the nature of the behavior setting.

Although the assistant was encouraged to engage patients in chiropractic conversation, it should not be construed that the waiting room was a center of constant ongoing focused interaction. The assistant was limited in his endeavors to sustain patients' attention by their receptivity. Tentative overtures were offered to patients with the hope of directing their attention to the topic of chiropractic care. However, if it was seen that an individual for one reason or another was reluctant to pursue the topic, it was tactfully avoided and the conversation directed to a general topic—or the exchange was terminated. The relative success of the assistant in this respect was both situational and problematical: it depended upon the number of persons in the waiting room, the nature and extent of their acquaintance, and the varying degrees of their chiropractic experience.

Supportive Others and the Inexperienced Patient

Approximately half of all the new patients observed during the time of the study were accompanied by one or more supportive others. Usually these persons were relations of the patient. As in a normal nondeviant medical setting it is quite common for parents to accompany a young child, an adult person to accompany spouses, or the young to assist the elderly. Unlike the traditional setting, however, interaction between the inexperienced patient and his supportive others was minimal. Evidence of mutual involvement was limited almost entirely to nonverbal indicators of togetherness, such as physical proximity, hand holding, exchange of reading materials, primary eye contact, and the taking of other similar interpersonal liberties.

When children were brought to the Clinic, they were required by their parents to remain seated and stern silence was usually demanded. Since literature and other forms of diversion for children were not available in the waiting room, discipline was sometimes a problem for parents concerned with maintaining proper appearances. Here, once again, a general lack of situational definitions was reflected by the parents' doubts concerning permissable lattitudes of behavior for their children. According to one parent:

When Stevie hurt his back, 'course we took him to the [medical] doctor right quick . . . but he never got all better. When a neighbor told us to try a chiropractor, we didn't know if they worked on kids. We called Dr. _____ [the Clinic] to find out if Stevie could come.

And again in a later conversation with the same couple, the wife apologized for the waiting room behavior of the son.

Stevie just won't stay still. I tried to get him to . . . but I guess he was nervous like we was. The girl [assistant] was so nice, she came out and talked to us and told Stevie about the couch [adjustment table], and well, it just made us feel better knowing we could all go in together, for one thing.

The presence of supportive others was reassuring and whenever possible the assistant would stimulate interaction between the patient and his supportive others thus promoting solidarity and relaxed confidence. Various conversational topics were pursued depending upon their appropriateness in the situation.

The subject of children and the problems of child-rearing provided natural opening gambits for the assistant. At times the practitioner's wife, when serving in the capacity of assistant, would bring her young child with her to the Clinic.[7] At those times when a child of a similar age was present, play would be encouraged in the waiting room. The children would be the focus of attention and the conversation would inevitably be steared in the direction of chiropractic and child care.[8] If possible, interaction was initiated among unacquainted persons who may have children of their own. Under ideal conditions, the initial encounter group, consisting of parents, children, and assistant was expanded to include several unacquainted persons in the waiting room.

Experienced Supportive Others

In an earlier study (Wardwell, 1951:233) it was observed that as a general rule it is favorable comments about the chiropractor from another person that persuaded the patient to try chiropractic and to select the particular practitioner that he does. This observation is supported in the present study. What was not indicated in this earlier work, however, is the significance of the knowledgeable supportive other in the behavior setting. In the Clinic it was not uncommon for the new patient to be accompanied by the

[7] It was not possible to ascertain whether this was a purposeful manuever or done simply for the sake of convenience.

[8] This is an important facit of chiropractic practice-building in that whole families are encouraged to come to the Clinic for periodic check-ups and adjustments "at reduced rates, of course."

referring significant other. Although many of these experienced supportive others were members of the immediate family, to be accompanied by a friend or acquaintance was not exceptional.

An established friendly relationship between the experienced patient and the assistant (and later the chiropractor himself) was characterized by a mutual openness (Goffman, 1963:131). The assistant greeted the new arrivals with a warm welcome and in turn was introduced to the prospective patient. The exposed position of the new patient provided the assistant with the license to approach him in a more direct fashion concerning chiropractic than was normally possible. Through the efforts of the assistant, the experienced patient was initially made the focus of interaction in the early stages of the encounter. The assistant could recall the experienced patient's success with chiropractic, or if possible, elicit a testimonial directly from him. The mutual regard and good will expressed in the encounter, combined with a fairly adequate supply of definitive ground rules supplied by both the assistant and the supportive other, served to sustain the new patient in his involvement in the chiropractic situation.

Supportive Interchanges

The sympathetic experienced patient was situationally supportive in two analytically distinguishable ways: first, he served to lend credence and support to the assistant's claims concerning the promise and effectiveness of chiropractic; second, he supplied the new patient with assurance in the setting, thus satisfying an implicit demand for a satisfactory definition of a deviant situation.

That the supportive other relieves the assistant of some of the "burden of proof" and the new patient of situational anxiety was illustrated by the following representative encounter. Howard K., a foreman and a regular chiropractic patient and William S., a laborer on the same crew, entered the Clinic late in the afternoon and were greeted by the assistant.

ASSISTANT: Hello Mr. K. Back so soon? Your regular appointment is scheduled for Thursday. Can't stay away, huh?

HOWIE: Nope. No trouble with me. Seems to be O.K. this week [referring to his arthritis]. But I got a man here who fell on the job this morning and can't get the tingle out of his leg. This is Bill S.

ASSISTANT: Please have a chair and I'll see if the doctor can examine you right away.[9] [Exits and returns immediately]. It will be just a few minutes. [She seats herself next to Howie, but addresses the new patient] I'm sure the doctor can help you. Sometimes these things can be cleared up right away. Right, Mr. K.?

HOWIE: Well, I'm working every day and feeling pretty good, that's for sure.

WILLIAM S., [visibly nervous] Well, I know I got something wrong with my legs and back, and if it's pinched nerves or something, well . . . [glancing at the assistant] I hope he doesn't mess it up worse."

9 In this instance, as in others, the assistant knew that the practitioner was unoccupied with other patients, and probably available. The new patient, especially if he or she is accompanied by a supportive other, is made to wait, the specific purpose being interaction engagement.

HOWIE: Come on. He'll adjust it back into place.[10] Listen, I've never walked out of here worse than when I come in. Usually a lot better. You'll probably feel as good as new tonight.

ASSISTANT: Well, we can't always tell about these things, but the doctor will know what's best for you. [to Howie] Thanks for bringing him in, Mr. K. I know we can help him. After all, hospital and drug bills [11] can run hundreds of dollars and you still won't be really well.

HOWIE: Yeah, for five bucks, what've you got to lose?

Although the above encounter was restricted to the three actors and could easily have taken place in the adjustment area, it was intentionally carried out in the waiting room as part of the standing pattern of behavior in the Clinic. Ideally such conversations took place in the presence of others with the hope of including them in the interaction or, at least, exposing them to it.

THE ADJUSTMENT AREA SUBSETTING

Chiropractic Teamwork

As noted, the practitioner and his assistants constituted a performance team in that they cooperated in the staging of a behavioral routine which served to supply the patient

10 The use of the term "adjust" indicates that this patient has begun to acquire at least a minimal chiropractic vocabulary.

11 As part of the training process, the practitioner admonished me to "never use the term 'medical' bills. The term 'drug' today means something bad, like 'drug user'."

with a specific and consistent set of definitions and expectations within the total configuration of the chiropractic setting. This cooperative teamwork was not immediately observable except in the most overt instances of normal role performance.

In a dramaturgical sense, the practitioner could have been viewed as not only the lead actor but also the behind-the-scenes director. He was primarily responsible for the appearance of the setting and behavioral regulation of the actors within it. For example, the assistant, while in the waiting room, by design had had the opportunity to "read" the patient, and at that time made a tentative judgment of the patient's receptivity to chiropractic health care.

The first specific evidence of behavioral collusion on the parts of the chiropractic actors in the setting was the exchange which took place between the assistant and the practitioner when the new patient was introduced into the adjustment area.

Often, just before the patient was taken in, the assistant would once again "see if the Doctor is free now," thus passing along any information about the patient in private. However, just as often, the assistant would take the patient directly to the practitioner with only a brief introduction.

In the event the assistant had no opportunity to talk to the patient, this would be indicated to the practitioner:

Dr. _____, this is _____. We've been so busy this morning, we haven't had much of a chance to get to know each other. Maybe you can make her feel welcome.

Lack of information about a new patient was deemed undesirable by the practitioner. Normally the approach taken by the practitioner when initiating the encounter depended primarily upon the cues he had already been given by the assistant, which were based on the waiting-room experience.

These essential but sketchy definitions of the patient were most helpful to the practitioner because he had learned from experience and training that patient attitudes toward chiropractic and the practitioner ranged from nervous anxiety to open hostility. Seldom did a new patient come to the Clinic with high positive expectations and confidence. How the practitioner handled this range of patient responses will be the focus of the next chapter.

The Presentation of the Chiropractic Self

Whether the patient entering the adjustment area was new or a regular, the practitioner welcomed him with easy warmth, inevitably indicating to the patient to "have a seat [at the table] and let's get to know each other a little," or, in the case of a regular, "let's bring ourselves up to date." Rarely was the patient directed immediately to the adjustment table except in the case of patients (almost always regulars) who demanded a quick adjustment because of time limitations or excessive pain.

With the exception noted above, all patients were engaged in conversation which was initiated, directed, and sustained by the practitioner. Whereas in the waiting room the assistant's task was to supply the patient with the assurance of an non-threatening situation, the practitioner in the adjustment area defined his own role in terms of supplying a specific set of definitions and ideas concerning the nature, purpose, philosophy, and promise of chiropractic. For the most part the practitioner assumed control of the interactional situation from the outset, leading and directing the flow of substantive topics.

I give him the works right off the bat . . . spell it out for him in black and white. If he's going to buy it, I've got to find out right away. I can usually tell in the first five minutes of talking to him and watching him how far I can go with some things [topics] and then I can kinda feel my way from there.

Opening statements dealt with the fundamentals of chiropractic and closely resembled the information which the patient had familiarized himself with by reading the brochures and pamphlets given to him in the waiting room. Besides supplying a degree of consistency in the behavior setting, it also allowed the practitioner to clarify any confusion or misconception held by the patient.

Beginning with the most general statements ("Chiropractic health care is as natural as blue skies and green grass!"), the conversation was systematically directed to the more specific. Emphasis on the naturalness of chiropractic was emphasized repeatedly: "Chiropractic enables the natural physiology of the body to take charge. Once we can get the natural energy within your body to flow like nature intended it to, we can get you well again."[12] One of the most obvious and repeated techniques of chiropractic salesmanship, evidenced in both the reading materials and in actual conversation, was the use of simple analogies:

[12] Note the repeated use of the plural "we." The patient is encouraged to believe that successful treatment is a matter of cooperative effort between doctor and patient, e.g., regular appointments.

You can understand that a house is in danger of collapse when its frame is out of line, or that the function of an automobile will prove defective and dangerous if its supporting structures are bent and distorted, and its movable parts out of alignment. Of course you can understand that bent and twisted body frameworks cause ailments throughout the entire body. But some people don't understand this.

In the attempt to anticipate an obvious question, the chiropractor eventually raised the problem of why there exists such misunderstanding of chiropractic. Stock explanations were offered such as a general lack of knowledge, the vested interests of powerful medical lobbyists and an erroneous faith in the germ theory of disease. It is at this point that the chiropractor attempted to rationalize, for the patient, the patient's curiosity, interest, and actual presence in the Clinic:

Mrs. R. [addresses her with the utmost seriousness and solemnity], you have no idea at this time just how fortunate you are having the courage to try chiropractic. If we could just convince more open-minded persons like yourself to come to us with their problems, much of the ignorance and suffering of the world would be solved. Thank you for having faith. [Standing up, he finishes.] Now let's get you well!

Before the actual examination procedure began, the patient was given ample opportunity to raise questions. The practitioner would insist that "it is especially important to get him to express his objections. I always hear him out. If I let him get on that [adjustment] table and he's full of negatives, he won't respond at all."[13]

13 By "respond" the practitioner was referring not just to a favorable acceptance on the part of the patient, but to an actual physical response, i.e., the "cure."

During the "warm-up" period in the adjustment area, the practitioner moved freely around the room taking advantage of the techniques of "stage business": pointing to wall charts and spinal displays, securing literature from the wall rack, making absent-minded adjustments on the adjustment table, and so forth. These movements all served to convey a relaxed and informal scene. The patient would be directed to a wall chart or to a small handwritten sign.[14]

After the patient was judged ready he was told, "Let's try out the table. We'll go slowly at first and you'll see that it's easy." When the adjustment table and the patient were lowered into a horizontal position, the practitioner gently placed his hands on the high-back, shoulder area of the vertebra. He often remarked to the new patient, "I can feel the tenseness throughout your body, especially your legs. Now I want you to relax and concentrate on your spine."

This observation and admonishment conveyed to the patient two things: (1) that the chiropractor was able to detect things throughout the body by a careful and probing examination of the spine, and (2) that the pattern of conversation had changed. Although the practitioner remained in control of the overall experience, the patient's *social* presence (as an interactional target) was no longer the center of attention.

Occult Involvement. At this point in the practitioner-patient encounter, the practitioner displayed what Goffman

[14] Repeated observations of the practitioner during this time revealed standing patterns of behavior which ordinarily would go unnoticed by the casual observer. For example, when the patient had been directed to the display skeleton for the purpose of informing him of the critical importance of nerve impingement, he was invariably referred to the small handwritten sign above it, which seriously proclaimed: "Accuse not Nature! She hath done her part; do thou but thine." This philosophy was "a natural for getting them on the table."

(1963:75–79) has termed an "occult involvement." He became engrossed in a specific and minute examination of the spinal column while at the same time displaying a marked inattention to the *social* presence of the patient.[15]

The practitioner, at the beginning of the actual physical examination, would tell the patient to remain quiet so that *both* could concentrate on the spine, thus indicating to the patient that he was, for the moment, "going away." Several moments would pass during which time the patient would ask the practitioner a simple question which may or, as was quite often the case, may not elicit a reply. Here was an activity which, it must be assumed, was meaningless to the patient, except in the gross sense of knowing that he was somehow being examined.

The aura of mystery was increased when the practitioner suddenly and without apparent reason would ask, for example, if the patient had experienced "any stomach trouble in the last few weeks: gas, indigestion, anything like that?"[16]

In most instances the patient would reply in the affirmative and at times would attempt to describe the complaint, only to be told, "Well, we can discuss that later, after your examination is completed." Several other specific inquiries

[15] This is a modification of Goffman's use of the term which designates "a kind of awayness where the individual gives others the impression . . . that he is not aware that he is 'away'." Further, Goffman uses it to refer to a form of negatively defined behavior—"unnatural . . . bodily activities" creating "disturbing impressions." The selection of the term occult rather than "away" seems appropriate. The practitioner was engaged in an activity, as mysterious as it may seem, as part of the practitioner's training and professionalism. "I didn't know what he was doing there, and I still don't. But after he told me what was wrong with me, I knew that *he* knew what he was doing!"

[16] These inquiries varied, of course, from patient to patient and from visit to visit. In most cases, however, they referred to the common complaints expressed by persons in everyday conversations. In most cases, for example, women were asked if they ever experienced difficulties during menstruation.

concerning the patient's recent or not so recent history of symptoms were made.[17]

While these questions could be interpreted as general inquiries concerning the patient's overall health, it was natural for the patient to conclude that there was some specific basis for each. This impression was reinforced by the following technique.

Just prior to each inquiry or observation the practitioner made it clear that he had found something which he had quite obviously been looking for. This was accomplished by a series of apparently non-communicative utterances:

Hmm . . . there seems to be a curvature here, so . . . let's see, there should be subluxation about here . . . no . . . uh, yes. Here, do you feel that: is that a little sensitive? Now tell me, have you had a recent fall or injury affecting your arms . . . ? Your right arm? Ah, yes. That's indicated.[18]

This form of examination procedure did have an im-

[17] It should be recalled from an earlier section (p. 73) that the assistant purposefully and tactfully avoided eliciting information concerning the patient's symptoms. The reason for this practice should be clear at this point: if the patient is allowed to know that the practitioner has been foretold of various complaints, the impact of these proclamations would be lessened or lost.

[18] It should not be construed that this procedure is fraudulent. Although the practitioner indicated to me that he sometimes guessed at probable common symptoms, he remained, as far as can be determined, convinced that he did indeed have the ability to accurately detect and assess the effects of vertebral subluxations.

It is not the purpose of this work to determine the quality of chiropractic care. The literature is replete with endless debate concerning the validity of chiropractic claims. Both sides involved in the argument cite research and authority. The controversy surrounding chiropractic may well be a political, rather than a scientific, debate. A similar point has been made regarding the marijuana issue in contemporary society: See Eric Goode's article, "Marijuana and the Politics of Reality" (1969).

pressive impact on most patients. Many saw the practitioner as having the power to see into the human body in what appeared to be a practical and straightforward way.[19] When the patient expressed surprise (and most did) at the chiropractor's observations, he was quick to follow up with the following comment:

Well, you see, this points up one of the major differences between the chiropractor and the medical doctor. When you go to the medical man you pay a lot of money so that *you* can tell *him* what's wrong with you. I feel that I should earn my money—[laughing] a lot less money, I should add—by telling you those things.

And further:

We're here not only to treat a specific problem but our goal is to do something about your total health. I know you didn't come here about a lot of those things [reviewing those symptoms which the patient has just acknowledged], but we're going to see a lot of improvement in things that you didn't know were wrong with you when you came in here.

Supportive Evidence: The X ray. The chiropractor saw the use of X rays as essential for three reasons: (1) they provided a source of immediate and substantial income; (2) once the patient had spent that sum of money he usually committed himself to at least a short series of appointments; and (3) the X rays offered much support to the statements made by the chiropractor concerning the patient's physical condition. If the patient queried, "Do I have to be

---

[19] This point is emphasized in McCorkle's short article (1961) dealing with chiropractic in rural Iowa.

X-rayed?," the reply was invariably, "Do you want relief or correction?" Very few patients refused.

After the X rays had been taken, the practitioner in most cases would employ the following procedure: (1) he reiterated the patient's condition; (2) he showed the patient the nerve chart on the wall, pointing to the patient's alleged difficulties; (3) the skeletal vertebral column was picked up and manipulated in various positions in order to demonstrate spinal distortions and subluxations; and (4) the X rays were shown.[20]

PRACTITIONER: You see, Mrs. M. [pointing to a specific area on the X ray], here is the source of a lot of your difficulty. A lot of that indigestion you have had stems from subluxations here . . . and here.

MRS. M.: Well, what about the arthritis in my hip? That's why I came here, you know.

PRACTITIONER: Please remember, chiropractic doesn't treat symptoms. Your spine [again pointing to the patient's X-ray] can suffer distortions at almost any point. Subluxation here between the second and third cervical [neck area] can bring about distortion even in the low back area.

MRS. M.: You mean indigestion can cause arthritis?

PRACTITIONER: Well, not exactly. All the unpleasant symptoms you feel are related since they all are produced by spinal

[20] This procedure is explicitly spelled out in a manual shown to me by the practitioner, James W. Parker, *Practice Building and Office Procedure*, "prepared especially for the Chiropractic Profession." Although the chiropractor was familiar with this and similar methodographic source material, he insisted repeatedly that the best procedure is that procedure which works for him (behavioral elements are unique to each behavior setting, as we have said above) and to follow a rigid plan in handling patients was construed by him to be "unnatural."

distortion. Our job, over the next few weeks—with your co-operation, of course—will be to correct this "dis-ease." After we have adjusted you on a regular basis, we'll take another series of X rays and you can see the progress we've made.

At this point the patient was instructed to return to the adjustment table. During the actual adjustment the practitioner directly discussed with the patient various specific spinal locations which he had previously identified on the X ray. The practitioner would systematically adjust the "sub-luxations," each being accompanied by an explanation of possible symptoms produced by each. A significant and unmistakable snap would be similar in effect to a popping of one's knuckles. Again, this reinforced the claims of the practitioner that there was indeed something there.

On occasion, some pain would be experienced, although this was rare for most patients of *this* practitioner. In the event of pain, the practitioner was quick to observe:

Say, that must have hurt a little. This is a little more serious than I thought. It means that you've suffered from this impingement a good while. Sometimes a fall or an accident in childhood can go unnoticed, but the longer the condition is left untreated the more troublesome it can be to correct it, not to mention your increased susceptibility to illness.

In order to allay any fears the patient would have of pain the practitioner would note that it would be possible to work on other parts of the spine, easier to adjust, the effect being to ease other more difficult parts. "We'll return to that spot later, after a few other easier adjustments, and you'll be surprised at how easy it will move."

Face Disengagement. Although the time spent on the actual adjustment could be quite brief ("A good chiropractor can adjust a known patient in two minutes)", the new patient spent on the average forty-five minutes in the adjustment area of the Clinic. Most of the time was spent familiarizing him with basic procedure and situational expectations, "dipping" him in chiropractic.

A significant part of the dipping procedure involved the rest period immediately following the actual adjustment. The rest period was significant in that it revealed the practitioner's concern for the quality of interaction which he sought to control:

It's a rest period in two ways. It *is* good for the patient to relax after the adjustment, but it also lets him just take a break, and think about things.

The following exchange took place between the practitioner and a young girl, Miss V., who, up to that time, had shown great anxiety and apprehension.

PRACTITIONER: Please stay in that position [prone, lying on her front with arms outstretched and her face placed between the two supportive cushions] and try to relax the body after an adjustment in order to let the spine respond.

Miss V.: I certainly feel relaxed. I could almost go to sleep.

PRACTITIONER: Well, don't do that, although most patients feel that way. Do you know what you're feeling? That's the natural strength which has been blocked for a long, long time. You're going to feel better when you leave here today, better than you've felt for a good while.

At times during this rest period the practitioner might have actually left the adjustment area, allowing the anxious patient a respite from the pressures of an uncertain social situation. But whether the practitioner was absent or present, the patient was allowed to break face contact and, in a sense, was permitted to be away from the necessity of what might have been uncomfortable, reciprocal, face-to-face interaction.[21]

ENCOUNTER TERMINATION: THE PATIENT'S "BURDEN OF PROOF"

As a preparatory gesture to terminate the adjustment area encounter, the practitioner would instruct the patient to "turn over now and relax for a minute while I get your file card and make some notes."

Upon his return to the adjustment area, the interaction pattern shifted abruptly. At this point the patient was given the responsibility of directing the flow of conversation.[22]

[21] At times during this rest period, patients were overheard talking to the practitioner about personal matters, e.g., a recent divorce, troubles at work or with children, and so forth. The practitioner would always listen sympathetically—sometimes taking notes for future reference—and occasionally making comments, not unlike the exchange which takes place in the office of a professional analyst. Some patients, it might be speculated, seek this kind of relationship with the chiropractor: a "poor man's therapy." A need for this kind of help, particularly for persons of the lower classes, has been suggested by Hollingshead and Redlich (1958); see also Redlich (1961).

[22] Again, I am not assuming intentionality here. The practitioner made it quite clear that this was part of his standard procedure. At times, when he was picking up an appointment card in his office, he would jokingly predict to me how a particular patient would react when given this burden of interactional responsibility.

Although the practitioner had attempted to anticipate the usual problems, questions, and concerns of the patient, he nevertheless encouraged the patient to express himself fully.

The specific content of this interaction was, of course, problematic and varied from patient to patient. Questions concerning fees and appointment dates were frequently forstalled "until we check with my assistant and the appointment book." Of central concern to the practitioner was the patient's general impression of chiropractic and his potential for future adjustments. Questions were answered and concerns countered with care and precision, the practitioner relying upon stock answers which would emphasize chiropractic philosophy.

As will be seen in the following chapter, the practitioner's "reading" of patient's receptivity and willingness to empathize with chiropractic philosophy, was essential to his procedure of typing patients. In some cases, patients were reluctant to pursue certain lines of discussion, and when this was the case, the practitioner, at times, would approach the topic from a different direction. For example, when attempting to elicit the patient's response to the notion of the Innate Intelligence within the human body, questions would be couched in terms either of the Deity or of Nerve Impulses —depending upon prior conversation.

It will be seen that the practitioner was not necessarily discouraged by a lack of response; some of his best regular patients—one of his patient types—were essentially non-communicative. Of greatest importance for the practitioner was the patient who responded negatively. Negative responses could center around a variety of subjects, although the most frequent objections were related to the practice of drugless therapy and the necessity of frequent and continuous appointments. These objections will be discussed in the chapter on patient typology which follows.

Fees and Appointments

The patient was led to the doorway of the private office where the assistant was waiting with the appointment book. The most immediate and practical concern for the practitioner at this time was convincing the patient of the necessity of regular and systematic appointments. If the patient had been X-rayed, the practitioner had learned from experience that in most cases the patient would return for at least one more visit. Again, depending upon the practitioner's reading of patient receptivity, various approaches to the problem of adjustment scheduling were suggested. Although the practitioner would have liked to have seen each patient two to three times a week, he realized the danger of losing certain patients if it was insisted upon. For the most part, the patients themselves ultimately determined the frequency and duration of the adjustment schedule.

Fee collection was routine. Most patients responded favorably to the relatively low cost per visit. The advantages of the prepay and family plans were pointed out as well as the possibility of insurance and medicare benefits. Once again the practitioner was aware of the patient's willingness to cooperate.

Although routine, the matter of fee collection was noteworthy since it clearly pointed out an example of the practitioner's methodographic technique. Drawing heavily upon suggestions for fee collection found in Parker's manual on office procedure (1965), the practitioner modified his collection methodology according to patient type.

As an example of the explicit instructions recommended by Parker, he suggests:

Don't be reluctant to say, "The examination, including all the pictures necessary, will be thirty-five (not dollars) and this will include (list the pictures individually) in addition to (some "extras" such as any X rays necessary under concentrated care you might find essential)." Incidentally, when quoting fees, mention the fee and then keep talking to enumerate what they will get for the fee. [Ibid:65]

The practitioner was observed using this approach almost verbatim on occasion, and other approaches were similarly employed as the situation demanded. The selection of methods depended primarily upon his prior methodographic training and past experience.

BACKSTAGE INTERACTION

In this section I am using a conceptual modification of Goffman's logical division of behavior settings into "front" (those features of the setting which are presented to the audience as part of the overall rhetoric), and "back" (that region which is inaccessible to the audience where persons can be off-guard with other actors and prepare for "front" performances). Earlier studies focusing upon this "front–back" dichotomy (see, e.g., Ball, 1967) have laid heavy emphasis upon the structural, spacial characteristics of behavioral regions while, for the most part, ignoring the temporal qualities of those regions.

In the Clinic, the backstage region has been described (p. 63, above) as being located primarily in the practitioner's private office. However, the main point here is that this region *came into existence* only at certain times, and to varying degrees. The implication is that, contrary to what the ecologists would emphasize, regions must be defined primarily in social rather than physical terms (see, e.g., Barker, 1968).[23]

The temporal relativity of regions[24] (subsettings) may be illustrated by the following observations made in the Clinic's backstage setting. First, patients, as a rule, were permitted into the private office at the termination point in the practitioner-patient encounter. (It will be recalled that the patient entered the office with the practitioner to discuss the matters of fees and appointment scheduling.) *At this point in time,* this region was not be thought of a backstage area; it constituted part of the front. Only at those times at which patients were not present—either no patients were in the Clinic or they were beyond hearing distance—did this region become backstage. Thus, this region existed only periodically.

---

[23] MacCannel (1973), in his study of tourism and social space—one of the most insightful works dealing with back regions to date—makes note of the social nature of regions. But even here, his treatment of them, particularly backstage regions, is worded primarily in physical terms.

[24] As used in this context the term "region" is a misnomer in that as normally defined it refers to a portion of territory or *space.* However, since the term has been used repeatedly and has become standard in the literature, to suggest an alternative would only serve to confuse more central issues.

Furthermore, there was a transitional quality of the back-stage region. As will be seen in the chapter which follows, certain patients became regulars in their visits over a period of time. Depending upon the practitioner's reading of the patient's honest sympathy toward chiropractic, he was allowed to participate to a greater or lesser extent in back-stage activity. My own personal experience as participant observer was illustrative.

Originally, as a patient, I was totally unaware of back-stage activity in the Clinic, although as a student of drama-turgical sociology, I recognized the probability of such interaction. Gradually as I became accepted by the practi-tioner and his assistant as good material for chiropractic training, more and more was revealed to me concerning his private (nonpublic) statements concerning his methodologi-cal and methodographical activities.

As MacCannel has indicated (although in a different context) it is useful to view the "front-back" dichotomy as ideal poles on a continuum.[25] Similarly, in the Clinic, regu-lar patients (including the writer) gradually moved *through time* from a position primarily "in front" of the performance to a privileged position "in back." Furthermore, it should be stated that although backstage, as defined here, existed periodically and transitionally, the following observations were recorded during those times at which the practitioner and his staff were confident of their privacy and my sin-cerity. "Insight, in the everyday, and in some ethnological senses of the term, is what is gotten from one of these peeks into a back region" (MacCannel, 1973:598).

[25] His continuum is discussed primarily in terms of physical (spacial) objects.

Backstage Methodography

One of the most significant observations to be stated concerning backstage conversation is the preponderance of time
spent on the topic of chiropractic. Reviewing the field notes,
rarely does there appear any record of subjects discussed
other than this.

Above, I have indicated that the practitioner was a "true
believer" in Eric Hoffer's sense of the term (1951). That
the topics of chiropractic history and philosophy were of
intensely personal, immediate, and practical (methodographical) concern for the practitioner was indicative of
this.

It must be admitted that my presence in the Clinic as a
trainee might have caused, at least in part, a disruption in
the normal conversational routine. However, for several
reasons, I felt this was not so. First, the practitioner was
engaged in similar conversations with several other sympathetic others, including his wife, other practitioners, regular
patients, and even casual acquaintances. "You never know
who you can turn on to chiropractic. If I live it, people are
impressed. I talk about it all the time to anybody who will
listen." Often these conversations were overheard by me,
the practitioner was either unaware of or unconcerned with
my presence.

Second, the practitioner, on two occasions during the
course of study, had invited fellow practitioners to his home.
These visiting chiropractors were accompanied by their
wives and children. When asked what they talked about, the
practitioner replied:

What else? Some of these guys I went to school with. This is what we do for a living. It's our lives. Sometimes we have study sessions and talk about lessons we had in school. We even review our old textbooks. It's a real party, everybody sleeping on the floor and all. It's a great life.

Third, when visiting other practitioners as a sympathetic patient (while seeking supportive data for this study), similar topics of conversation were not uncommon.

It was from the conversations that took place in the Clinic between the practitioner and myself (in many cases they resembled lectures with question and answer periods), initiated and sustained by the practitioner, that the material for the second chapter in this study was gathered. Little effort on my part was needed to elicit historical and philosophical information, it was an integral part of backstage conversation.

Performance Disruptions and Remedial Methodography

The practitioner was beset with numerous difficulties in the Clinic. He earned a modest income, and felt it did not reflect his actual professional potential. Moreover, the chiropractor who had formerly occupied the building and was now leasing the office space, the adjustment table, and X ray equipment to the practitioner, was having financial troubles of his own. On several occasions they quarreled over rental payments, and threats were made to evict the practitioner.

Consequently, the practitioner was sensitive to the responses of some of his problem patients and often expressed uncertainty as to his capabilities as a professional. These and other problems were discussed and analyzed during those periods of backstage privacy.

Advice from Supportive Others.   Being alone in the Clinic except for his staff and not having immediate recourse to the council and advice of another nearby professional ally the practitioner felt it necessary, at times, to place long distance telephone calls to Dr. Sid (see p. 43 above). He had met this chiropractor while attending Palmer College and knew him personally. Unfortunately, I was never able to witness these conversations and must rely solely upon what the practitioner related to me concerning the subjects discussed; however, there is no reason to believe that any information was altered or deleted.

When attempting to support and encourage the practitioner, Dr. Sid would cite examples of other chiropractors, including the early forefathers, who experienced "tremendous difficulties when trying to carry the [chiropractic] message to the people." The practitioner was urged to recall the basic principles of chiropractic, which deal with the positives and negatives of human existence as they become manifest in the human body. Chiropractic, he was reminded, has as its immediate purpose the elimination of physical negatives. This principle can and must be applied to the matter of daily living:

He told me to "eliminate the negatives from my practice." I've got to locate the sources of trouble in the Clinic and do something about them. These trouble spots can cause negative attitudes for me and when I have a bad attitude it can cause more troubles. He [Williams] said that we [himself and the staff] have to figure out where things might be going wrong and do something about them. . . . We've got to learn from the experience and mistakes of others who've been through this before. . . .

This kind of advice, coming from a prominant spokesman of chiropractic, supports the contention that history and philosophy are of paramount methodographic importance for many if not most chiropractors.

To use the practitioner's term, these conversations were "pep talks" and presumably would apply to any chiropractor. "Of course, he [Dr. Sid] has never been in this Clinic and doesn't know exactly what's wrong, but he gives good advice just the same."

Dr. Sid, along with other spokesmen of chiropractic, sponsored several meetings around the country during which they offered advice concerning the practicalities of running a clinic. Practitioners spent hundreds of dollars to attend these meetings and, according to editorials in chiropractic journals, most meetings realized high attendance. Thus, the practitioner had available to him explicit methodographic techniques designed to ameliorate various difficulties as they might occur.

Flexibility in one's procedural method was often emphasized. According to a passage, pointed out to me by the practitioner, from Parker's *Manual*:

Look for successful methods, not a retirement plan. Be ambitious, not ultraconservative. Develop growth-potential, not self-depreciation. Make a list of your strengths. . . . Possess a BIG-THINKER'S vocabulary, not a defeatist's slang . . . GO FIRST CLASS. Pick your environment . . . .

Analysis of the Physical Setting.   From time to time, the practitioner would consider making changes in the arrangement of the waiting-room furniture, his private office, or the adjustment area. For example, new stage props were considered. "You know, maybe we ought to put a Bible in the waiting room. We could turn it to a passage on 'the laying on of hands,' or something like that."[26]

Although few changes were actually made during the time of the study (except for the handwritten signs), the topic arose on numerous occasions. New ideas were sought by examining pictures of other chiropractic clinics as depicted in the practitioner's trade magazines, which he regularly received. Following a basic plan learned while a student at Palmer, the practitioner had rearranged the furniture of the office during his first days in the Clinic. Accordingly, he felt reluctant to risk major changes which might have unexpected results or be viewed unfavorably by his professional superiors.[27]

Analysis of Standing Behavior Patterns.   As in the case of physical arrangements in the Clinic, the practitioner expressed reluctance to alter, in any substantial way, those patterns which were recommended that he use in his training in office procedure.

[26] This idea was eventually rejected, the practitioner explaining that he didn't feel competent to cope with theological questions that might possibly arise from the presence of a Bible.

[27] As an example of this last point, the practitioner at one time seriously considered selling health foods as a sideline in the waiting room. He intended to let his wife or myself be in charge of sales. This idea was also rejected since he was unsure of how Dr. Sid would respond. "He's a 'straight,' you know, and he doesn't believe in mixing anything with the truth of chiropractic."

Predominant standing behavior patterns (e.g., the "first come, first served" method of receiving patients, the method of introducing patients into the adjustment area, the X-ray procedure, fee collection and appointment scheduling, and encounter termination techniques) underwent slight modification, if any, during the time of the study. However, as in the former instance, several alternative procedures were considered from time to time. (Virtually all aspects of the behavior setting at one time or another were methodographically examined with the hope of uncovering some hidden difficulty.)

Analysis of the Performance Team. One of the most obvious examples of methodographical activity involved the analysis of the cooperative teamwork of the staff. The practitioner was especially aware of and concerned with the coordination of his staff and the manner in which they (himself included) presented and sustained a consistent front through their personal actions toward their patients. Once again, my experience as assistant-in-training is illustrative.

Part of my backstage training consisted of the appropriate use of "stage talk." "Don't come on too strong with words; you can scare people sometimes by talking over their heads; use words like 'honesty,' 'sincere,' 'love,' things like that. Leave the big stuff to me."

The specific meanings of chiropractic terms were discussed in great detail. "We've got to agree on things. If you tell a patient one thing and I tell him another, he gets the idea we don't know what we're talking about."

The problem of presenting a consistent front to the audience was a major concern for the practitioner. Of special importance for him was the manner in which his assistants prepared the patient for his entry into the adjustment area particularly for the first time. He discussed and rehearsed with us the manner in which we should defer to his knowledge and experience in matters directly pertaining to chiropractic. The matter of avoiding eliciting information from the patient concerning his overall health has already been discussed, and the examination for that technique made apparent. On this he commented backstage:

It's really impressive when I tell the patient what's wrong with him. It's not the kind of thing that happens when he goes to a medical doctor. Don't spoil the show for me by getting him to tell you his entire case history.

Audience Analysis: Treatment of the Absent.   A fourth subject of methodographic activity, closely related to the last, dealt with the techniques of reading patients.

A major premise of interaction theory refers to the persistent and ongoing attempts of human social actors to determine the perceptions, conceptions, and intentions of all significant others. Although it is a basic human activity, persons are, most of the time, unaware of this process.

Conversely, the practitioner was not only intensely aware of this activity, but was quite concerned with his accuracy in determining patients' definitions of the situation and of himself. "It's very important for me to figure out how a person is going to respond to chiropractic and to me."

Much backstage conversation was directed toward various means of assessing patient responsiveness. The importance of engaging patients in conversation prior to and after his experience with the practitioner in the adjustment area was stressed. The practitioner, while forming his own impressions of patients as the result of his own contact with them, relied heavily upon the interpretations of his staff. We were told to

. . . watch carefully for any sign of [the patient's] confusion or trouble [dissatisfaction] and let me know about it right away so we can do something about it. Get friendly with them, but be careful. Some people don't like it when you get too personal, especially when they've got something to gripe about.

As Goffman has indicated:

[W]hen members of a team go backstage where the audience cannot see or hear them, they very regularly derogate the audience in a way that is inconsistent with the face-to-fact treatment that is given to the audience . . . . Sometimes, of course, the opposite of derogation occurs, and performers praise their audience." [1959:170–171].

It was during periods of private backstage discussion in the Clinic that the practitioner and his staff exchanged views of patients and patients became typed or previous typifications were modified.

In the following chapter, several examples will be cited which pertain to the practitioner's reading of patients' definitions of the situation. Although the practitioner depended primarily upon his own interpretations of the responses of various patients, at times he would indicate some confusion. At these times he would seek our interpretations and we would discuss at length these persons. Ultimately, there would emerge a classification which would provide the practitioner with a plan of action toward that patient in future encounters.

A careful examination of the procedure involved in the typing of patients is discussed in the following chapter.

CHAPTER FIVE

A Chiropractic Patient Typology

The main concern of this chapter is the elucidation of the practitioner's typing of virtually all patients who entered his Clinic. His reasons for doing so are seen through the labeling approach to social deviance, this approach being based on and a direct outgrowth of the symbolic interactionist tradition. The practitioner is viewed *not* as a passive recipient of a deviant label, but rather as a possessor of a considerable degree of power within the behavior setting.

The labeling perspective has recently been criticized for its failure to adequately take into account the labelee's power to effectively handle the deviant label accorded him by society at large. Schervish (1973) has extended this criticism on two grounds: the assumed passivity of the labelee,[1] and a tendency to focus upon the individual rather than on the group as the unit being labeled.[2] Traditionally,

---

[1] See, e.g., Goffman (1961), Scheff (1964, 1966), Schur (1965), Erickson (1964, 1966), Cicourel (1968), Matza (1969), Duster (1970), Cicourel and Kitsuse (1963).

[2] See, e.g., Sykes and Matza (1957), Goffman (1961), Freidson (1965), Turk (1966), Scheff (1968), Erikson (1968), and Klapp (1962).

the sociology of deviance (and the labeling perspective may be included) has focused upon the pariahs of society, i.e., those persons whom obviously violate the norms of the social order and are handled accordingly. Although the notion of secondary deviance (the process by which the labeled person begins to take on as part of his self-conception those attributes of the label) has been introduced,[3] the individual, even in this context, is seen as a passive recipient, responding in a more or less deterministic way. Schervish views this tendency in the labeling approach as being antithetical to the Meadian heritage upon which the perspective is founded:

The Meadian perspective enables sociologists to designate the process of becoming deviant (cf. Matza, 1969) rather than merely to assert that "mind" or "personality" or some other intervening unknown or "black box" acts as deterministic transmitter or forces, impinging upon the actor and making him deviant. [Schervish, 1973:47]

The present study of a chiropractor as a marginally deviant individual affords the chance to assess the assertively active performance of the labelee in a behavior setting of his own design and control, i.e., the setting allows him the maximum freedom to structure the ongoing interaction which takes place within it. The chiropractor is viewed not as a passive agent in the Clinic, blindly responding to the social forces which surround him, but as a volitional actor in the sense of having a considerable command over the situation.

[3] Lemert (1967).

Furthermore, the practitioner, having had a body of formal training in his vocation, was supplied with a highly significant professional reference group by which he was enabled to critically assess, modify, and rationalize his performance in a variety of situations. Whenever difficulties or doubts arose concerning practical problems in the Clinic, help was readily available from this reference group.

The association to which he belonged, the ICA, would supply him with philosophical, financial, and legal support if the need arose. Thus, the chiropractor was further viewed as possessing a considerable degree of power—in the sense that he was not powerless to negotiate the social reality within the Clinic's setting.

THE DEVIANT (CHIROPRACTOR) AS LABELER

A second major source providing impetus to the development of the labeling perspective (in addition to Mead's contribution) is the work of Alfred Schutz.[4] A predominant theme in his work is that social reality for all human beings is a matter of classification of everything that one comes into contact. Indeed, this is the basic notion underlying the term label in that it allows social groups to classify, and therefore make understandable, various forms of behavior which violate certain values. By labeling inappropriate forms of behavior and thus placing them in some definitive

[4] For a succinct discussion of the theoretical convergences giving rise to the labeling perspective, see Schur (1971:115–158).

context, plans of action become possible providing orientation in problematic situations.

Previous studies utilizing this perspective have focused almost entirely upon the phenomenon of labeling as it is carried out by those persons who represent powerful elements in the social order. However, the possibility of viewing the labelee as participating in the same sort of activity has been neglected.

The practitioner engaged in a form of social psychological activity which is rendered understandable when viewed in the labeling context. In other words, the practitioner as labelee, may now, quite properly, be viewed as *labeler*.

Certain forms of behavior occurred in the Clinic which the practitioner deemed inappropriate or deviant; accordingly, persons engaged in these behavior patterns were labeled (typified), thus allowing the practitioner various plans of action.[5] The question of his *power* to apply the labels will be discussed in the sections which follow.

THE CHIROPRACTOR AS MARTYR

The preceding chapters have dealt almost exclusively with the presentation of the chiropractor's self-image in a situation which has been shown to be at least marginally deviant. The practitioner himself readily admitted his devi-

---

[5] Although it was not discussed in this context, Becker's analysis of the professional dance musician suggests the same phenomenon: musicians type some audience members as "squares." As a symbolic expression, "such words enable musicians to discuss problems . . . for which ordinary language provides no adequate terminology" (1963:143).

ant status and, in a very real sense, took pride in it in the same sense that a religious martyr takes pride in and consoles himself with his martyrdom. The practitioner confided in me one day during a backstage conversation:

You know, if chiropractic wasn't considered a kind of "far out" thing, it wouldn't be half so much fun. I really think that if everyone thought chiropractic was O.K., it would be just another way to get well. A lot of us through the years have suffered because of the law and a bad name and things like that, but that's the reason why a lot of us keep working so hard to bring people the truth.

The practitioner encountered daily information, both through the media and personal relationships, which defined his profession as a deviant health care practice. He recognized and readily admitted his deviance, and yet, in the face of all opposition, maintained that he was right in the sense of possessing "the truth about the natural way of the body."

He saw himself as deviant in a formal sense in that he knew he violated established health care practices. Yet, by appealing to "higher loyalties" (Sykes and Matza, 1957), namely the natural and Eternal Truths of chiropractic philosophy and those who espouse it, he sought to neutralize the label in order to present to himself a consistent and acceptable self-image. Thus, he was free to engage in a form of behavior which was manifestly deviant yet did little damage to his self-esteem.

Any self-image, deviant or otherwise, has as its ultimate source the perceived reflected intentions of significant others. As described below, the practitioner had the ability, to a considerable extent, to manipulate the quality of his clientele in order to create for himself the most favorable audience for his professional activity.

THE PROBLEM OF PATIENT RESPONSE

During the course of his practice, the practitioner encountered a range of patients who responded to chiropractic in various ways, from more or less open receptivity (these were rare) to overt hostility. Both the practitioner and his patients usually experienced an incomplete biographical sketch of each other, especially in the initial encounter. As Glaser and Strauss (1964:669–679) have noted, this situation necessitates the "bracketing" of the encounter into an immediate situational awareness context out of which biographical knowledge of each other is constructed relative to that point in time and space.

Ideally, this allows each actor (in this case, both the practitioner and the patient) to determine the latitudes of permissible behavior, provides a basis for determining the actions of the other towards himself, and also provides a set of more or less acceptable responses to those actions.

THE CRITERIA OF PATIENT ACCEPTABILITY [6]

As indicated in the previous chapter, the practitioner perpetuated a front designed to accomplish two ends: (1) it presented to patients and to others a situational orientation

[6] These criteria, as summarized here, have not been assumed but were elicited from the practitioner in the course of numerous backstage

within the setting, and (2) it provided a means of systematically assessing patients' response and receptivity to that setting. Among the criteria which the practitioner utilized in accomplishing the latter objective were: (1) the degree of behavioral involvement in the setting, e.g., how relaxed the patient felt, how much anxiety concerning the adjustment and X-ray procedure and/or cost was shown, and how much freedom of physical movement was evidenced; (2) the depth of philosophic conversation, e.g., the patient's willingness and ability to ask questions of an abstract nature concerning chiropractic; (3) the extent of occult involvement, i.e., the patient's willingness to discuss covert perceptions of the negative effects of the "dis-ease" and, later, of the positive, ameliorative effects of the adjustment; (4) the extent to which the patient was willing to share the practitioner's views of the medical establishment; (5) the extent to which the patient's attitudes were modifiable, i.e., the patient's willingness to change his mind concerning prejudices toward chiropractic; and (6) the possibility of commitment to chiropractic health care as a permanent way of life.

Admittedly these criteria may overlap, but for the most part, according to the practitioner, they supported and complimented each other in the sense that taken together, they provided a means of assessing the overall expressions "given" and "given off" (Goffman, 1959:2) by the patient toward the practitioner, the Clinic's setting, and chiropractic in general.

---

conversations. Their significance was validated by direct observation, non-directive commentary by the practitioner, and by the subsequent interviews with him during the last days of the study.

THE TYPOLOGY

As indicated above, the following typology was based primarily upon the interpretations of the practitioner. It should be noted, however, that the categories were not completely his own, in that a chiropractic publishing company (operated by Dr. Sid in conjunction with the ICA) had printed a brochure describing three patient types. Dispensed to patients in the Clinic, this one-page foldout was entitled, "There Are 3 Types of Patients: Which Type Will You Be?" The brochure was illustrated by caricatures which were supposed to show, by means of facial expressions (frown, half-smile, grin), the typical responses of patients. The first type, because he feels so improved after the initial treatment, stops going to the chiropractor before he has been totally cured. The second type discontinues chiropractic treatment because he does not feel better after the first few treatments. The third type is restored to good health because, although he may feel better, he continues treatments until "the chronic nerve interference is removed."

The practitioner did not merely adopt this simple classification, but embellished and modified it in a fashion relative to his own practice and patient experience. The categorical names, with the exception of the regular patient, were not normally used in the presence of patients, but were used extensively in backstage conversation, thus enabling the performance team to share a common set of definitions and orientation to patients.

The practitioner prided himself on his ability to type a

The One-Timer or the One-Shot Patient

patient "five minutes after he walks in the door," and this ability was most evident with those patients *labeled* as one-timers.

The practitioner was quick to respond to the opening remarks given voluntarily or through questioning which would indicate the patient's prejudices toward chiropractic. Often a patient would enter the Clinic with a specific complaint and seek quick recovery on a short-term basis of two or three visits. This type of patient often had seen a chiropractor before and for one reason or another, had experienced some degree of success. For example, a member of the coaching staff of a local team entered the office one afternoon holding his back and walking in a stooped position. He was shown into the adjustment area, as in the case of all emergency patients. Walking immediately to the adjustment table, he demanded, "Let's get this over with quick. I've got to be back in twenty minutes. I sure as hell can't run around in this position."

The practitioner began the adjustment process immediately. Although several attempts were made to engage the coach in conversation, all failed, except for noncommital statements. After the adjustment was completed, the patient arose and handed the practitioner a five-dollar bill and departed with a hurried promise to return "when I have the time to do it right."[7]

[7] In McCorkle's study of chiropractic in rural Iowa (1961), this

After he had left, the practitioner commented to me "Sure I straightened him out, but I didn't really help him. He might be back in a few months when it goes out again. You can't count on his kind at all."

Also included in the one-shot category are those patients who, for the most part, failed to significantly respond to the practitioner's rhetoric. Most persons would listen with courtesy to the practitioner's presentation from beginning to end. Some patients offered little response in an observable fashion except in the everyday pleasantries of any formal encounter between unacquainted persons. The practitioner would approach such patients during the encounter with a variety of performances, seeking what he referred to as an opening, sometimes with little success.

At times the practitioner expressed frustration ("Sometimes I get so damn mad I feel like telling them to stop wasting my time and theirs, but of course you can't do that"), although he considered his time well spent if for no other reason than that of income. "When they don't respond . . . it's both bad and good, depending on how you look at it. They don't usually kick when I bring up the X ray and the fees . . . and you know the money isn't bad for an hour's work even though I might not see them again."

If a patient refused to respond overtly, the criteria for patient acceptability was for the most part inapplicable in that the reaction was neutral. The patient presented no opportunity for biographical construction; he remained a

---

patient response was typified as the norm, since persons in that geographic area were defined as "practical people who seek an immediate, simple solution to their problems." This observation is obviously an oversimplified one, as is demonstrated in the sections which follow.

nonentity, indicating neither positive nor negative attitudes toward chiropractic, the behavior setting, or the practitioner himself.

Since the one-shot patient provided little basis from which the practitioner could evaluate his behavior in the setting, he had a tendency to lapse into a standard presentational routine. At the termination point, for example, he would assume what might be described as a quite formal, even brusk, attitude toward the patient. He was never impolite, but he would dismiss the patient with tact and little or no attempt to persuade the patient to continue treatment.[8]

During the course of this study every attempt was made to initiate conversations with patients who had clearly been designated as falling into one category or another.

This was done in order to assess their differential responses to the treatment they received during their session in the adjustment area. A typical one-timer patient response was reflected in the comments of Mr. Y., a retired worker who had come in to "see about my health." At no time did he voice a specific complaint, enter into sympathetic interaction with the practitioner, or elaborate extensively upon his experiences in the adjustment area except for the following observations:

ASSISTANT (MYSELF): Well, what do you think of chiropractic?

[8] Once the researcher became aware of the practitioner's conception of the one-timer as a patient type, the practitioner was timed by stopwatch technique in the initial encounter with the patient. After two or three minutes, he would sometimes return for a file card or some other reason and would indicate to me his perceptions concerning the patient. It was noted that although the average time spent with all other *new* patients was approximately forty minutes, the time spent with the one-shot patient was approximately twenty-five minutes.

MR. Y.: I learned a lot about it, I guess.

ASSISTANT: I see the Doctor has you down for another appointment.

MR. Y.: Yeah, well, if I'm not feeling any better I guess I'll be back; but if it clears up I probably won't.

ASSISTANT: You know, it's like the Doctor says, if you feel better then that's the time to continue adjustments. It means you're responding to the treatments and it's a good way to stay well.[9]

MR. Y.: Well, I guess that's right. We'll see . . . .

Mr. Y. never returned. Some weeks later, the practitioner was asked why.

PRACTITIONER: I told you he wouldn't be back. I could see that right away. When he came in, I ran him through the procedure and got some X rays, but I'll never use them.

ASSISTANT: I noticed he didn't stay as long as some of the other new patients. Did he have to leave early?

PRACTITIONER: No, I don't think so, but I didn't waste much time with him either. I mean, why should I? He wasn't coming back.[10]

9 While participating in the role of assistant the researcher was careful at all times to present to patients the verbal rhetoric specified by the practitioner as "part of your job."

10 According to W. I. Thomas (1932), if actors define a situation as real in a specified manner, future events in the ongoing situation will reflect those prior definitions. Similarly, Merton (1957) has termed this phenomenon a "self-fulfilling prophecy." If the practitioner in this case gives off the impression that he doesn't expect to see the patient again, this expectation may become shared by the patient, thus fulfilling the one-shot prophecy. When the patient did indeed fail to return, this served to reinforce the practitioner's conviction that he had the ability to accurately read each patient typically. This notion of defining situations as real is just as applicable to other patient types.

The Problem Patient: Deviance Within a Deviant Setting

Although the practitioner did seem to have the ability to predict the behavior of many patients, he was often wrong. Occasionally a patient who had been typified as a one-timer did return to the Clinic much to the surprise of the practitioner. Many patients who eventually were typed as problems followed this pattern. Quite often the patient, although he had missed the scheduled appointment, would return to seek relief from a recurring problem at various and unpredictable times.

Typically the patient would resist the practitioner's efforts (now renewed) to convince him of the benefits of regular chiropractic care. At one extreme, the patient would remain noncommital, while at the other, open antagonism and even hostility might be expressed.

It was not possible to delineate a specific set of behavioral characteristics to describe the problem patient. A problem patient was identified as such due to his inability to meet the criteria of patient acceptability as defined by the practitioner. Whereas the one-timer typically remained passive in his non-acceptance of chiropractic and/or the practitioner, the problem patient responded negatively.

One conversation which was recorded extensively in the field notes exemplifies the negative and disruptive comments of patients labeled extremely problematic. Miss A., a middle-aged teacher who had seen the practitioner irregularly four times over a six-month period prior to this visit, complained of a backache and general fatigue. When the practitioner saw her name on the waiting list, he grimaced, rolled his eyes toward the ceiling, and said to me, "Well dammit, here we go again!" The following are excerpts from their conversation in the adjustment area:

PRACTITIONER: Here are the X rays we took, let's see . . . uh . . . five weeks ago. It's been a long time. All we can do is hope for the best. Why don't we check it [indicating the adjustment couch]?

MISS A.: Well, you certainly don't sound very encouraging.

PRACTITIONER: Miss A., I'm going to be very honest with you. There isn't very much I can do for anybody unless they take my advice and begin a series of regular appointments. We really don't work miracles here—although some people are convinced we do—but we do allow the body to correct itself over a period of time the way God intended it.

MISS A.: Let's leave God out of it if you don't mind. I don't think we speak the same language. [Placing herself on the adjustment table, she insisted:] Well, let's get this over with. I'm in a hurry.

At this point the practitioner commenced his technique of suggesting possible symptoms of dis-ease while carefully examining her spine. Several attempts were made to this end, all of which were responded to negatively.

MISS A. [quite exasperated]: No, no! None of those things. I feel fine. It's my back that hurts, not my head! Why don't you work on my back and leave the rest of me to a doctor who knows what he's doing.

PRACTITIONER: Did you read *any* of the material I gave you the last time you were in? . . . Well, I wish you had. It would make things a lot easier.

The practitioner began the adjustment accompanied by standard, under-the-breath comments to himself.

MISS A.: What? What's that you said?

PRACTITIONER: Oh, nothing. It just helps me to concentrate on your condition. It wouldn't mean much to you anyway . . . .

When the adjustment was completed, the practitioner motioned to Miss A. to be seated at the small table.

MISS A.: No, I'm late as it is. How much do I owe you this time?

PRACTITIONER: The standard fee. Five dollars.

MISS A.: You must be a millionaire. Your adjustment didn't take five minutes.

Without pausing at the door of his private office, Miss A. hurriedly handed him the fee as she was leaving, giving him no chance to pursue the possibility of a future appointment. Said the practitioner to me, after she had left, "That's that! Good riddance."

The above example illustrates the failure to meet most, if not all, of the criteria for patient acceptability. Although most problem patients did not exhibit such an extreme negative reaction, this pessimistic and antagonistic attitude was not uncommon.

Ironically, although the problem patient actually brought more business to the Clinic than, say, the one-timer, the practitioner frequently returned the antagonism, even to the point of open rejection. For example, one day he was overheard commenting to a patient who had insisted on combining chiropractic and prescription medicine:

How do you expect me to get you well if you insist on poisoning yourself [with "drugs"]? If you feel that the medical doctor is doing more for you than I am, then you are wasting your time here. You might as well not come back.

In sum, the problem patient was disruptive in his behavior in three ways: (1) his attendance was irregular, thus violating one of the tenets of chiropractic philosophy and procedure; (2) his overt behavior within the behavior setting was unpredictable, thereby preventing the practitioner from constructing a systematic and reliable biography of the patient, and determining a course of action in the setting; and (3) his behavior served to threaten the practitioner's self-conception.[11]

Rationalizations for Patient Rejection. After the author became aware of the practitioner's tendency to select his clientele in the fashion described above, the practitioner was asked, "How can you justify driving away patients when you repeatedly tell me of the difficulties of practice-building? It seems you are defeating yourself." The practitioner offered the following explanations:

1. *Long range—outside the Clinic:* "A bad patient can really hurt your business. He may bring in a few dollars, but it's not worth it. When he goes home with bad attitudes and talks to friends and neighbors about it, it can really hurt. . .∴. I've even lost some regulars because they've been turned off by a friend of theirs."

[11] As Goffman has noted, " . . . the individual may deeply involve his ego in his identification with a particular part, establishment, and group. . . . When a disruption occurs, then, we may find that the self-conceptions around which his personality has been built may become discredited" (1959:243).

2. *Immediate—inside the Clinic*: "You've seen me take patients out of the waiting line? Well, those are usually problem patients who like to talk about their complaints about me. I can't let those troublemakers spread that gossip in the waiting room. I once had a fight going out there between a problem and a regular. I haven't seen either one since."

3. *Personal*: "When I have a run-in with one of them [problem patients], it spoils my whole day. It's like Dr. Sid says, you've got to get rid of the negatives. If all my patients gave me trouble like some of them do, I don't think I could take it. . . . The regulars make it all worthwhile."

The Regular Patient

Whereas the problem patient was irregular in attendance, unpredictable in his behavior, and threatening to the practitioner's self-image, the regular patient, conversely and ideally, evidenced none of these undesirable characteristics.[12]

The practitioner noted two principal sources of regular patients: transfer patients—patients who had been seeing another chiropractor—and converts.

Transfers[13] usually presented little difficulty for the prac-

[12] Although a wide variety of patients may become regulars ("a 'regular' is made, not born"), at least half of the patients identified as such by the practitioner were either retired persons of either sex or housewives. Although it is not within the intended scope of this paper to assess the empirical characteristics or psychological attitudes of patients from an outsider's point of view, this clearly is an area for study. See Schmitt (1974).

[13] It will be recalled that there was another chiropractor in the same community, but he was of the mixer variety. Depending upon the patient's prior exposure to chiropractic, he would select one or the other, in many cases, by following the recommendation of his previous chiropractor. Straight chiropractors recommend other straights, and mixers, other mixers. Both have membership lists (ICA, ACA) for this purpose.

titioner in that his situational rhetoric and adjustment procedure was representative of other straight chiropractors.[14] Most entered the situation with a clear-cut set of definitions and experienced little difficulty in adjusting to the surroundings.

Those persons with whom the practitioner ultimately realized success in the conversion process were those persons whom in most cases he had identified previously, sometimes after only one or two sessions, as showing good potential. Occasionally, a one-timer who was misjudged would become fairly regular, but this was rare. Never once, during the course of the study in the Clinic, was it observed that a problem patient became a regular.

Supportive Others and the Regular Patient. Regulars were accompanied to the Clinic by supportive others much more often than either of the other two patient types discussed above. It was quite common for the supportive other (or others, in the case of families) to become converted, and become regular as well. These persons at times would request that their appointments be set up to coincide with each other.

Furthermore, persons previously unacquainted, would sometimes establish friendships within the Clinic and would also arrange their appointments together. This was supported and encouraged by the practitioner who saw this as beneficial both to his patients and to his business.

[14] Although no attempt is made to demonstrate the representativeness of the Clinic relative to other chiropractic offices, support for this statement is provided by (1) the practitioner's own testimony, (2) the author's own impressions based upon visits to other chiropractic clinics, and (3) the responses of patients who had previously been exposed to chiropractic elsewhere.

Eliciting Testimonials.   At times, when the practitioner would observe that several fairly regular patients (who may have been more or less acquainted) happened to be in the office at the same time, he would suggest that "we all get together in the adjustment area to get to know each other a little better."

During such a session (usually brief—five to ten minutes —and quite casual) the practitioner would attempt to elicit personal testimonies concerning success with chiropractic. Also, patients would be asked their opinion concerning articles appearing in chiropractic magazines and journals. Such give-and-take sessions were conducted with informality, each patient participating freely with little or no prompting by the practitioner. These discussions at times would focus upon a wide variety of topics, mostly dealing with personal chiropractic success, chiropractic philosophy, the problems of everyday living, and the solutions to such problems. The practitioner was quick to emphasize the simple, natural logic of chiropractic, "which is really much more than just a way of keeping healthy, it's a whole way of life."

Booster Patients.[15]   A regular patient who becomes convinced that he has experienced success ("It really seems to be doing me some good"; "It's miraculous! I've never felt better.") would often voluntarily promote chiropractic. These boosters were encouraged to spread the word and

[15] The term "booster" was not coined by the practitioner but is found throughout chiropractic publications. Parker, for example, in his practice-building manual, discusses various techniques for utilizing the potential of boosters. For example, " . . . make certain to introduce and encourage conversation between regular and prospective patients if the regular is a booster-type patient" (ibid.:68).

bring in new patients. Quite often this was done despite the fact that no financial renumeration was offered.

Ample supplies of free literature were provided for these patients and the practitioner considered the money well spent. Indeed, several new patients were brought to the Clinic through these boosting efforts during the course of the study.[16]

Recruits. Chiropractors occasionally encounter a patient (usually a regular) who expresses such interest in and commitment to chiropractic that he seeks to convince this individual of the advantages of chiropractic as a profession. This is not an uncommon practice for either straight or mixer chiropractors. Recruitment pamphlets and short application forms were observed in all chiropractic offices visited. As far as can be determined, the chiropractor receives no reward, either from his professional organizations or the colleges, for the recruitment of new persons into the profession. His efforts were apparently strictly voluntary.

One of the main reasons the researcher realized success in achieving a considerable involvement in the behavior setting and success as a participant observer was the practitioner's conviction that I was "choice material for Palmer College of Chiropractic." By showing enthusiasm and sympathetically supporting his excitement about his profession, I established and sustained a relationship with the practi-

---

[16] Before the state laws licensing chiropractic were put into effect, advertising in the various forms of mass media (now illegal) was a common means of acquiring new patients. Large advertisements promoting clinics were placed in town newspapers. These ads consisted primarily of testimonials from satisfied patients, a picture of the booster being predominant.

tioner not unlike that which existed between himself and several other strongly supportive patients.

This chapter has been devoted to processes by which the practitioner (1) *perceived* the varieties of patient response, (2) *assessed* these responses in light of his past experiences and the biographical source material he had gathered for each patient, (3) *typified* each patient thus allowing him a course of action in future encounters, and, finally (4) *adjusted* his own behavior in light of these categorical definitions.

The ultimate consequence of this overall process was to *eliminate* those persons who persisted in responding unfavorably to the practitioner's efforts to present a satisfactory chiropractic front and to *convert* those others who had demonstrated sympathetic inclinations.

Thus, the notion of impression management and the techniques normally associated with it may be enlarged to include a technique which heretofore has received little recognition: one can present and sustain an image of oneself by adjusting both appearance and actions, *and managing the composition and overall "quality" of the audience.*

CHAPTER SIX

General Review, Statement of Contributions, and Suggestions for Future Research

Chiropractic is the largest and most influential of the competing health care practices in the United States. Labeled deviant by at least six formal, rule-making, and sanctioning bodies, chiropractic, as a profession, has struggled for recognition by and approval from American society at large. A radically unique explanation of the origin and nature of disease, coupled with an internal division or conflict within this occupational group (Leis, 1971), has hindered its professional image.

The present study has focused upon one chiropractic clinic in an attempt to examine the consequences of what has been referred to as the marginally deviant status of the practitioner who ran it. Although no major assumptions were held prior to the research, it seemed obvious that what took place in this setting was different from what one would normally expect in an establishment medical doctor's office. Of central concern were the various points of view and

sic

social meanings held by the various actors within this behavior setting: the practitioner himself, his regular full-time assistant (his wife), and the numerous persons who came to the Clinic as patients.

Utilizing the symbolic interactionist stance, coupled with the sensitizing concept of the behavior setting, and employing the methodology of participant observation, this study has sought to provide a body of empirical data not characterized by the bias often shown in the so-called objective approach which is normally employed in sociological studies of deviant behavior. By seeking out actors' definitions of the situation by a careful examination of their observable actions, including their interactions, and observing how they create and maintain rationalizations for those actions, the object has been to specify interactional patterns within that behavior setting.

Being an ethnographic account, this study has not had as its purpose the support or rejection of any theory or derived hypotheses put forth before or developed during the study. As a result, the most systematic means of evaluating the success of such an endeavor is to summarily review contributions to the sociological enterprise in the area of deviant behavior in general and to the study of the chiropractor in particular.

First, as indicated, although chiropractic as a profession has received some attention by sociologists (Wardwell, 1951; McCorkle, 1961; Mills, 1966; Sternberg, 1969; Leis, 1971; Schmitt, 1974), no work has been done on the everyday *behavior* of the chiropractor himself in the realities of a social situation. Being a representative of one of the most influential competing health care systems in the United

States, the chiropractor, as a social actor, has deserved this type of attention.

Although the present work has focused upon one practitioner in one clinic, it has been shown that there is every *sic* reason to believe that this Clinic is not unlike others, especially if they are operated by straight chiropractors. For such reasons this study should shed further light on the profession as a whole.

Second, this study has added to the comparatively recent *methodological* efforts to supply data on social deviance, i.e., that methodology which demands the gathering of data within the actual ongoing situation. Traditional objective methods have recently been criticized for their tendency to gather and remove data from the realities of everyday social phenomena. Statistics and removed-from-the-scene reports do not reflect the natural context of deviance.

The methodology utilized in this study represents an attempt to convey the behavioral actualities of a chiropractic practitioner, his staff, and his patients as actors within an unconventional behavior setting of the practitioner's own design.

A third contribution is the manner in which the task of presenting a *history* and general review of substantive literature was handled. Traditionally, this necessary task has been approached, again, from an objective stance. This has been seen to have its limitations in that it does not reflect the perceptions and conceptions, which are inextricably bound together, of the actors in the world of their everyday lives.

A major assumption, based upon the premises of symbolic interactionism, is that the social actor relies upon *past* learned experiences (in this case, primarily the practitioner's formal and informal training and his experiences in the Clinic) in order to (1) perceive, evaluate, and modify his behavior in *present* situations, and (2) orient his behavior in such a way as to prepare himself and others for imagined *future* events.[1]

Thus, by presenting a general history, philosophy, and socio-legal status of chiropractic from the point of view of the central figure in the Clinic, it is seen to be directly applicable to the understanding of his actions, i.e., *his* explanations and rationalizations of his own actions, the actions of others, and the interactions which took place between them.

Fourth, the present study has attempted to define a set of delimiting and directional guidelines within which the notion of a *behavior setting* becomes operationally heuristic. Drawing upon an earlier work done in the field of ecological psychology, the chiropractic clinic in this study was defined in terms of a total configuration delimited by spacial and temporal barriers. Also included were physical objects and standing patterns of behavior relative to those objects.

For the ecological psychologist, these spacial and temporal characteristics are, in a sense, given. In the present work, they are seen as being socially relative to the situation as it emerges *through* time (as distinct from existing *in* time). An example of this last point, it will be recalled, was

---

[1] This statement, it should be noted, is an oversimplification of Mead's argument in which he asserts that even present behaviors are in actuality future-oriented.

For an elaboration of this particular philosophical point, see Mead (1932).

the practitioner's awareness of these situational qualities and his attempts to modify them as he problematically conceived of the necessity for doing so. In other words, the behavior setting was, at least, always potentially modifiable according to his situationally relative definition of that setting. From a symbolic interactionist view, the physical setting and the social setting are inseparable: one cannot be considered without the other.

A fifth contribution, closely related to the discussion above, is the empirical demonstration of *methodographic activity* on the part of the principal actor in the behavior setting. Buchler has stated that all persons engaged in professional activities before a public ("audience," in Goffman's dramaturgical terms), methodographically assess and modify their appearance and behavior ("presentation of self"), i.e., their methods of impression management. Clearly, this is consistent with the interactionist's position that social actors possess the capability of modifying their courses of action relative to their changing definitions of the situation. As seen in the previous chapter, the practitioner was clearly cognizant of differences among patients in terms of a variety of responses to him and to chiropractic in general. In light of these perceived differences among patients, he methodographically assessed and modified his methods of self-presentation.

Not only was this concept useful in the understanding of much of the practitioner's behavior in the Clinic, but the empirical evidence of this phenomenon in an actual situation provides at least partial support for Buchler's claim for trans-situational applicability. Thus, it appears to be a viable conceptualization.

A sixth contribution, and possibly the most significant finding of the entire study, necessitates a careful reexamination of what is seemingly an implicit assumption held by those researchers utilizing the labeling approach to deviant behavior: the labeled person is seen to be a relatively powerless individual, responding passively to the label as it is applied by other individuals who possess social power. (This point is well-documented by Schervish in the article mentioned in Chapter Five.)

It is obvious that the practitioner in this study did possess a considerable degree of social power. It was power not in the sense normally thought of when considered as a coercive force, but power in the sense that he was able to manipulate the composition of the audience directly confronting him. In other words, he had the ability to (1) eliminate certain patients who persisted in their definitions of him as a "quack" by labeling them, in turn, deviant in the sense that they failed to meet his standards of patient acceptability, and (2) having been trained in the techniques of salesmanship, he could present an acceptable front to other patients, thus assuring their return to the Clinic. By eliminating some and securing the allegiance of others, he could create for himself a fairly stable and satisfying standpoint from which to see himself as a competent professional (George Herbert Mead's role-taking process).

Although other attempts have been made to demonstrate the deviant's attempt to neutralize the deviant label (e.g., Sykes and Matza, *Techniques of Neutralization* (1957)), the question of whether or not an individual labeled deviant could possess the ability to manipulate the audience (the labelers) has not been considered. Perhaps similar examples can be found in which the deviant possesses this power to control the make-up of the audience immediately confronting him (e.g., the ivory tower college professor). If so, a comparison of the techniques employed by these diverse marginally deviant persons would be valuable for future research.

Certainly, another area which demands closer attention than it has received in the limited research seen so far pertains to the socioeconomic characteristics of persons who seek out the services of marginally deviant health care practitioners (see Schmitt, 1974). The question of why these persons deviate from the norm of seeing the establishment medical doctor when physical problems arise remains to be answered. Furthermore, the psychology of conversion to a deviant health care service is even more of a mystery. Hopefully the present work will add insight to questions dealing with chiropractic and/or similar forms of marginal deviance.

Chiropractic Act of Louisiana

ACT No. 39

House Bill No. 712.   By: Messrs. Stephenson, Breaux, Gunter, R. S. Thompson, Scogin, Strain, Wilson, Rice, Toca, Jones, Triche, LeBlanc and Baker and Mrs. Johnson and Senators W. D. Brown, C. M. Brown and Dykes.

AN ACT

To amend Title 37 of the Louisiana Revised Statutes of 1950, by adding thereto a new chapter, to be designated as Chapter 36 thereof, comprising R.S. 37:2801 through R.S. 37:2818, both inclusive, relative to the practice of chiropractic and the regulation and licensing of chiropractors in this state, to create and provide with respect to the Louisiana Board of Chiropractic Examiners, its membership, powers, duties and functions; to provide with respect to fees, internship, and licenses; to provide an exemption from license taxes; to provide with respect to unlawful practices; to provide that said board's authority shall be exclusive; to provide penalties for violations; to provide for the rights and authority of licensees; to define terms, to provide requirements and procedures for licensing of applicants; to provide special provisions, to provide for the applicability of the Act; and to generally and specifically provide with respect to all matters related to all the foregoing.

Be it enacted by the Legislature of Louisiana:

Section 1. Chapter 36 of Title 37 of the Louisiana Revised Statutes of 1950, comprising R.S. 37:2801 through R.S. 37:2818, both inclusive, is hereby enacted to read as follows:

CHAPTER 36. CHIROPRACTORS

§2801. Definitions

As used in this chapter:

(1) "Board" means the Louisiana Board of Chiropractic Examiners.

(2) "Licensed chiropractor" means persons licensed under the provisions of this chapter.

(3) "Practice of chiropractic" means the holding out of one's self to the public as a chiropractor and as being engaged in the business of employing objective means to ascertain the alignment of the vertebrae of the human spine, including the use of analytical instruments of demonstrable efficacy for the purpose of analysis; and the practice of adjusting or manipulating the vertebrae and adjacent tissue for the purpose of correcting interference with nerve transmission and expression, on a person other than himself; and such exercise, external application of heat or cold and recommendations relative to personal hygiene and proper nutritional practices for the rehabilitation of the patient. The practice of chiropractic does not include the right to prescribe, dispense or administer medicine or drugs, or to engage in the practice of major or minor surgery, obstetrics, acupuncture, X-ray therapy or radium therapy.

§2802. Board of chiropractic examiners

A. The Louisiana Board of Chiropractic Examiners is created. It shall be composed of eight members who shall be appointed by the governor. Six of the members shall be chiropractors licensed under the provisions of this Chapter, who have been continuously engaged in the practice of chiropractic in this state for at least five years, and two of the members shall be practicing physicians licensed by the Louisiana State Board of Medical Examiners; provided, however, that the initial members required to be chiropractors shall be persons who are eligible to be licensed under the provisions of this Chapter.

The initial members shall be appointed within thirty days after the effective date of this Chapter to serve for terms of one, two, three and four years, as designated by the governor at the time of appointment. Thereafter, the terms of members shall be for four years each or until the successor of each member takes office.

B. Every chiropractor appointed to the board after the initial appointments shall be a licensed chiropractor under the provisions of this chapter.

C. Any vacancy occurring in the membership of the board, except by expiration of the term, shall be filled for the unexpired term in the manner provided in Subsection A of this Section.

D. The governor may remove any member for misconduct, incompetence or neglect of duty, after he has given the member a written statement of the charges against him and has afforded him an opportunity to be heard.

E. The governor shall issue each member a certificate of appointment. Within thirty days after the date of his appointment and before commencing the discharge of his duties, each member shall subscribe to the oath for public officials, which shall be deposited with the secretary of state as provided by law.

F. Each member shall serve without compensation, but shall be paid, out of the moneys credited to the board as provided by R.S. 37:2809(B), for actual travel and clerical and incidental expenses necessarily incurred while engaged in the discharge of his official duties.

§2803. Organization of board; quorum; meetings; records; rules and regulations

A. Within fourteen days after the appointment of all its initial members the board shall hold a meeting for the purpose of organization and shall elect from its membership a president, a vice president and a secretary-treasurer, each of whom shall serve a term of one year or until the successor of each is elected. Thereafter, the board shall annually and in like manner elect its officers.

B. The board shall meet on the second Monday in April and October of each year and at any other time the board deems necessary, at a time and place designated by the president. Special meetings may be called by the president upon giving at least seventy-two hours' notice sent by registered or certified mail to the post office address of each member of the board and to persons who previously have indicated that they have business before the board.

C. A majority of the total membership of the board shall constitute a quorum for the transaction of business. However, the granting, suspending or revoking of a certificate or license to practice chiropractic shall require the affirmative vote of at least five members.

D. The board shall keep a record of its proceedings and a register of all applicants for certificates or licenses, which shall contain the name and location of the institution which granted the applicant a diploma, the date granted, and information as to whether a license has been granted or refused. The record and register shall be prima facie evidence of all matters recorded therein.

E. The board shall adopt and promulgate rules and regulations to govern its actions and to provide for the enforcement of the provisions of this Chapter, pursuant to the provisions of R.S. 49:951, et seq.

§2804. Powers and duties of board

A. The board shall be the sole and exclusive authority in the state of Louisiana to issue licenses to practice chiropractic and to administer the provisions of this Chapter.

B. The board shall have authority to examine for, grant, deny, approve, revoke, suspend and renew the licenses of chiropractors and shall review applications for licenses at least once a year. It may conduct hearings on charges for the revocation or suspension of a license.

C. The board shall initiate an action for the prosecution of any person who violates any provision of this Chapter and may apply to any court having jurisdiction for an injunction to restrain and enjoin violations thereof. It shall keep a record of all proceedings relating thereto.

§2805. Requirement for license; penalty; qualifications; examinations; issuance of license.

A. No person shall engage or attempt to engage in the practice of chiropractic in this state who has not been licensed in accordance with the provisions of this Chapter.

Whoever violates this Subsection shall be fined not more than three hundred dollars or be imprisoned for not more then* three months, or both, and each day a violation continues shall constitute a separate offense.

B. The board shall license as a chiropractor and issue an appropriate certificate to any person who files with it a verified application therefor, accompanied by such fee as is re-

---

*As it appears in the enrolled bill.

quired by R.S. 37:2809, together with evidence, verified by oath and satisfactory to the board, that he:

(1) is at least twenty-one years of age;

(2) is a citizen of the United States;

(3) is of good moral character;

(4) is a high school graduate;

(5) has completed at least sixty hours of course work at a college or university of liberal arts or science which, at the time of attendance thereof, was fully accredited by a nationally recognized accrediting agency;

(6) has graduated from a chiropractic school or college which, at the time of attendance thereof, was accredited by the Association of Chiropractic Colleges or the Council on Chiropractic Education, or their successors, and approved by the board, and which was based on at least four thousand resident classroom hours;

(7) has passed an examination given and graded by the board, with a score of at least seventy-five percent, in the following subjects, namely, (a) anatomy; (b) physiology; (c) hygiene; (d) nutrition; (e) pathology; (f) symptomatology; (g) chemistry; (h) principles and practice of chiropractic; (i) x-ray procedure, interpretation and the effects of x-ray on the human body; (j) bacteriology; (k) public health, including communicable and contagious diseases; (1)* neurology, and (m) physical diagnosis.

If the applicant fails to pass the examination, not more than two examinations in the subjects failed shall be allowed without additional fee, upon request therefor by the applicant.

C. After investigation of the application and other evidence submitted, and not less than thirty days prior to the examination, the board shall notify each applicant that the application and evidence submitted for consideration is satisfactory and accepted, or unsatisfactory and rejected. If an application is rejected, the notice shall state the reasons for such rejection.

D. The examination shall be given annually at such time and place and under such supervision as the board may determine, and specifically at such other times as, in the opinion of the board, the number of applicants warrants.

The board shall designate the place of examination in advance.

E. The board shall keep written examination papers, an

---

*As it appears in the enrolled bill.

accurate transcript of the questions and answers relating to oral examination, and the grade assigned to each answer thereof as part of its record for at least two years subsequent to the date of examination.

§2806. Interns; qualifications, requirements

A. Pending issuance of license by the board, any graduate chiropractor who possesses a diploma from a college of chiropractic accredited by the Association of Chiropractic Colleges or the Council on Chiropractic Education, or their successors, and approved by the board, and who complies with the provisions of R.S. 37:2805(B)(1) through R.S. 37:2805 (B)(6), may intern for not to exceed one year with any chiropractor licensed under this Chapter at the office of said chiropractor and under his personal supervision. Prior to the end of the internship period the intern must successfully pass the examination provided for in R.S. 37:2805(B)(7). If the intern fails three or more of the subjects on the examination, he thereafter is prohibited from interning in this state.

B. A chiropractic intern may practice only while the supervisory, licensed chiropractor with whom he is interning is physically in the same building and office with him.

§2808. Reciprocity licenses

The board may grant a license to practice chiropractic without examination to a chiropractor who complies with the same or equivalent requirements as are set forth in R.S. 37:2805 and who is licensed by another state.

§2809. Fees

A. The board shall fix and collect uniform fees which shall not exceed the following amounts for each type of fee and which shall not be refundable:

(1) Application fee for license to practice chiropractic .... $ 50.00

(2) Certificate of internship .... $ 25.00

(3) For issuing duplicate of any certificate or license .... $ 5.00

(4) Certificate for annual renewal of license ...... $ 50.00

(5) License to practice chiropractic .... $ 50.00

(6) License by reciprocity $150.00

(7) Inactive license renewal .... $ 25.00

B. All fees received by the board and all fines collected under the provisions of this chapter shall be transmitted to the state treasurer, who shall place them in a special fund to the credit of the Louisiana Board of Chiropractic Examiners. The board shall have authority to expend the moneys in said fund for the operating expenses of the board and for other expenses incurred in the administration and enforcement of this Chapter.

§2810. Renewal of license

Beginning with the calendar year 1975, each license to practice chiropractic in this state shall be renewed annually on or before October 31st of each year, upon payment of the renewal fee prescribed in R.S. 37:2809 and the presentation to the board of a certificate showing satisfactory attendance of at least one two-day chiropractic educational seminar or convention approved by the board. However, for good and reasonable cause, the board may waive the convention or seminar requirements.

§2811. Recordation of license

A. Every licensee shall record his license with the clerk of court for the parish in which he practices, and until recorded, the holder thereof shall not be entitled to practice chiropractic in this state.

B. The clerk of the district court for the parish where the license is recorded shall keep an index of such licenses. The clerk may charge one dollar for the recordation of each license.

§2812. Statistical certification

Chiropractors shall observe and be subject to all federal, state, parish and municipal regulations with regard to public health and all other information required by law as coming within their knowledge. Chiropractors shall sign certificates and statements pertaining to public health insofar as they relate to chiropractic, but nothing in this chapter shall be construed to permit any chiropractor to execute or register certificates of birth or death.

§2813. Other annual license taxes not required

Licensed chiropractors and interns shall not be required to pay any annual license fee or tax except as provided in R.S. 37:2809 (A).

§2814. Waiver of renewals while in the military service

The board shall waive the requirements of R.S. 37:2810 for any chiropractor licensed under this chapter while in the military service of the United States or any of its allies, upon notification by the licensee to the board.

§2815. Display of license or certificates

Licenses and renewal certificates issued under the provisions of this chapter shall be conspicuously displayed in the principal office of the licensee.

§2816. Suspension or revocation of license; causes; hearing

A. After notice and an opportunity for hearing, the board may suspend or revoke any license or certificate issued to any chiropractor for any of the following causes:

(1) Conviction of a crime.

(2) Fraud, deceit or perjury in obtaining a diploma or certificate of licensure.

(3) Habitual drunkenness.

(4) Habitual use of morphine, opium, cocaine or other drugs having similar effect.

(5) Deceiving or defrauding, or attempting to deceive or defraud the public.

(6) Obtaining or attempting to obtain payment for chiropractic services by fraud, deceit or perjury.

(7) Incompetency, gross negligence, or gross misconduct in professional activities.

(8) Intentional violation of federal, state or municipal laws or regulations relative to contagious and infectious diseases or other public health matters.

(9) Violation of provisions of this chapter relating to the use of x-ray machines and procedures.

(10) Engaging in practice of the healing art beyond the scope of the practice of chiropractic, as defined in this chapter.

(11) Professional association with an unlicensed practitioner which in any way furthers or promotes the unlicensed practice of chiropractic.

(12) Holding out to the public the ability to cure a manifestly incurable disease or guaranteeing any professional service.

(13) Prescribing, dispensing or administering any medicines or drugs.

(14) Solicitation of professional patronage by advertising or any other means whatsoever, other than by conservative announcements of entry into or change of location of practice and/or association, professional business cards, and commercial or professional directory listings, which notices, cards and listings shall be limited to the name, specialties, if any, addresses and telephone numbers of the practitioners involved, in a brief statement of the purpose of the notice or listing.

(15) Using the title "Doctor," "Dr." or its equivalent, without using the term "chiropractor," or its equivalent, as a suffix or in connection therewith, under such circumstances as to induce the belief that the practitioner is entitled to practice any portion of the healing arts other than chiropractic as defined herein.

B. Nothing in this Section shall be construed to prevent a licensed practitioner from mailing educational material to his patients or the dissemination of educational material approved by the board or by chiropractic societies or associations.

§2817. Special provisions; persons practicing chiropractic on June 1, 1974; persons having passed National Board of Chiropractic Examiners examination; members of armed forces

A. Any person who was engaged in the practice of chiropractic in Louisiana on June 1, 1974 may apply to the board for a license. The application must be postmarked no later than sixty days after the first meeting of the board and shall be accompanied by the application fee required by R.S. 37: 2809(A)(1) and by certified proof of graduation from high school, or the equivalent thereof, and of graduation from a college of chiropractic accredited by the Association of Chiropractic Colleges or the Council on Chiropractic Education, or approved for purposes of membership by the American Chiropractic Association or the International Chiropractic Association, or graduated from a Louisiana chiropractic college and approved by the board. Upon compliance with this Subsection:

(1) An applicant who has practiced chiropractic in Louisiana for at least eight years when this Chapter becomes effective shall be granted a license without examination, provided he has not failed a board examination or had his license revoked in another state prior to beginning practice

in Louisiana. In the event of such failure of examination or revocation of license, he shall be entitled to take the examination required for applicants under Paragraph (2) of this Subsection.

(2) Applicants who have practiced chiropractic in Louisiana less than eight but more than two years shall be entitled to take an examination in x-ray procedures, physical diagnosis, and public health, including communicable and contagious diseases.

(3) Applicants who have practiced chiropractic in Louisiana less than two years must meet the requirements of R.S. 37:2805 (B) except 37:2805 (B) (5).

(4) Applicants described in this Subsection who have passed the examination given by the National Board of Chiropractic Examiners may take the examination provided for in Paragraph (2) of this Subsection in lieu of the examination required by R.S. 37:2805 (B) (7).

B. The requirement of R.S. 37:2805 (B) (5) is waived for any Louisiana resident who on the effective date of this chapter is attending a chiropractic school or college accredited by the Association of Chiropractic Colleges or the Council on Chiropractic Education, or their successors, and approved by the board.

C. Members of the armed forces of the United States or its allies who were practicing chiropractic, as herein defined, in Louisiana at the time of their induction and who at that time possessed a valid diploma from a school or college of chiropractic which is accredited and approved by the Association of Chiropractic Colleges or the Council on Chiropractic Education or their successors and approved by the board, shall be considered as having been in the state prior to the effective date of this chapter and may comply with the provisions of Subsection A of this section not later than sixty days after separation from the armed forces, and upon notification by the board of eligibility to practice chiropractic under the provisions of this Chapter, shall be issued a license upon payment of the fee required by R.S. 37:2809 (A) (5) hereof.

D. X-ray; use; procedures; prohibited uses

A chiropractor licensed under this chapter is entitled to utilize x-ray procedures for the sole purpose of chiropractic analysis. Such x-ray procedures shall be administered with efficient exposure techniques and optimal operation of radiation equipment in order to minimize the amount of and repetition of x-ray exposure to which a patient is subjected during such analysis.

Such procedures shall not include radio-therapy, fluoroscopy, or any other form of ionizing radiation, except x-ray, which may be used only for the purpose of chiropractic analysis. X-ray film shall not exceed 14 by 36 inches in size. The womb of pregnant females shall not be exposed to x-ray radiation.

A chiropractor utilizing x-ray procedures must comply with the provisions of R.S. 51:1053 et seq. and the regulations promulgated in accordance therewith.

Chiropractors shall retain all x-ray films taken in the course of their practice, together with the records pertaining thereto, for a period of three years.

The requirements and limitations herein set forth with respect to the use of x-ray procedures by chiropractors shall be enforced by the board.

§2818. Exceptions and rights

A. Nothing in this chapter shall be construed as conferring upon the holder of a license to practice chiropractic the right to practice medicine and surgery as a physician or osteopathic physician as defined by statute nor shall said holder be considered a licensed physical therapist as defined by statute.

B. This chapter shall not be applicable to licensed doctors of osteopathy.

C. Every person duly licensed and registered pursuant to this chapter shall have the right: to practice chiropractic as defined herein; to use the title "Doctor of Chiropractic" or "D. C."

Section 2. If any provision or item of this Act or the application thereof is held invalid, such invalidity shall not affect other provisions, items or applications of this Act which can be given effect without the invalid provisions, items or applications, and to this end the provisions of this Act are hereby declared severable.

Section 3. All laws or parts of laws in conflict herewith are hereby repealed.

Approved by the Governor: June 26, 1974.

A true copy:

WADE O. MARTIN, JR.
    Secretary of State.

The Thirty-Three Principles
of Chiropractic Philosophy

1. THE MAJOR PREMISE
    A Universal Intelligence is in all matter and continually gives to it all its properties and actions, thus maintaining it in existence.

2. THE CHIROPRACTIC MEANING OF LIFE
    The expression of this intelligence through matter is the Chiropractic meaning of life.

3. THE UNION OF INTELLIGENCE AND MATTER
    Life is necessarily the union of Intelligence and Matter.

4. THE TRIUNE OF LIFE
    Life is a triunity having three necessary united factors, namely, Intelligence, Force, and Matter.

5. THE PERFECTION OF THE TRIUNE
    In order to have 100% Life, there must be 100% Intelligence, 100% Force, 100% Matter.

6. THE PRINCIPLE OF TIME
    There is no process that does not require time.

7. THE AMOUNT OF INTELLIGENCE IN MATTER
    The amount of intelligence in any given amount of matter is 100% and is always proportional to its requirements.

8. THE FUNCTION OF INTELLIGENCE
   The function of intelligence is to create force.

9. THE AMOUNT OF FORCE CREATED BY INTELLIGENCE
   The amount of force created by intelligence is always 100%.

10. THE FUNCTION OF FORCE
    The function of force is to unite intelligence and matter.

11. THE CHARACTER OF UNIVERSAL FORCES
    The forces of Universal Intelligence are manifested by physical laws; are unswerving and unadapted, and have no solicitude for the structures in which they work.

12. INTERFERENCE WITH TRANSMISSION OF UNIVERSAL FORCES
    There can be interference with transmission of universal forces.

13. THE FUNCTION OF MATTER
    The function of matter is to express force.

14. UNIVERSAL LIFE
    Force is manifested by motion in matter; all matter has motion, therefore there is universal life in all matter.

15. NO MOTION WITHOUT THE EFFORT OF FORCE
    Matter can have no motion without the application of force by intelligence.

16. INTELLIGENCE IN BOTH ORGANIC AND INORGANIC MATTER
    Universal Intelligence gives force to both organic and inorganic matter.

17. CAUSE AND EFFECT
    Every effect has a cause and every cause has effects.

18. EVIDENCE OF LIFE
    The signs of life are evidence of the intelligence of life.

19. ORGANIC MATTER
    The material of the body of a "living thing" is organized matter.

20. INNATE INTELLIGENCE
    A "living thing" has an inborn intelligence within its body, called Innate Intelligence.

21. THE MISSION OF INNATE INTELLIGENCE
    The mission of Innate Intelligence is to maintain the material of the body of a "living thing" in active organization.

22. THE AMOUNT OF INNATE INTELLIGENCE
    There is 100% of Innate Intelligence in every "living thing," the requisite amount, proportional to its organization.

23. THE FUNCTION OF INNATE INTELLIGENCE
    The function of Innate Intelligence is to adapt universal forces and matter for use in the body, so that all parts of the body will have co-ordinated action for mutual benefit.

24. THE LIMITS OF ADAPTATION
    Innate Intelligence adapts forces and matter for the body as long as it can do so without breaking a universal law, or Innate Intelligence is limited by the limitations of matter.

25. THE CHARACTER OF INNATE FORCES
    The forces of Innate Intelligence never injure or destroy the structures in which they work.

26. COMPARISON OF UNIVERSAL AND INNATE FORCES
    In order to carry on the universal cycle of life, Universal forces are destructive, and Innate forces constructive, as regards structural matter.

27. THE NORMALITY OF INNATE INTELLIGENCE
    Innate Intelligence is always normal and its function is always normal.

28. THE CONDUCTORS OF INNATE FORCES
    The forces of Innate Intelligence operate through or over the nervous system in animal bodies.

29. INTERFERENCE WITH TRANSMISSION OF INNATE FORCES
    There can be interference with the transmission of Innate forces.

30. THE CAUSES OF DIS-EASE
    Interference with the transmission of Innate forces causes incoordination of dis-ease.

31. SUBLUXATIONS
    Intereference with transmission in the body is always directly or indirectly due to subluxations in the spinal column.

32. THE PRINCIPLE OF COORDINATION
    Coordination is the principle of harmonius action of all the parts of an organism, in fulfilling their offices and purposes.

33. THE LAW OF DEMAND AND SUPPLY
    The Law of Demand and Supply is existent in the body in its ideal state; wherein the "clearing house," is the brain, Innate the Virtuous "banker," brain cells "clerks," and nerve cells "messengers."

References

Ball, Donald W. 1967. "An Abortion Clinic Ethnography." *Social Problems*, 14 (3): 293–301.

Ball, Donald W. 1973. *Microecology: Social Situations and Intimate Space*. New York: Bobbs–Merrill.

Barker, Roger G. 1968. *Ecological Psychology: Concepts and Methods for Studying the Environment of Human Behavior*. Stanford, Calif.: Stanford University Press.

Becker, Howard S. 1963. *The Outsiders*. New York: Free Press.

Becker, Howard S. and Blanche Geer. 1960. "Participant Observation: The Analysis of Quantitative Field Data," in Richard Adams and Jack J. Preiss (eds.), *Human Organization Research*. Homewood, Illinois: Irwin.

Berger, Peter L. and Thomas Luckman. 1966. *The Social Construction of Reality*. New York: Doubleday.

Biemiller, Andrew J. 1970. AFL–CIO report submitted to U.S. Senate Finance Committee: "Fact Sheet." (September 15.)

Blumer, Herbert. 1969. *Symbolic Interactionism: Perspective and Method*. Englewood Cliffs, N.J.: Prentice-Hall.

Buchler, Justus. 1961. *The Concept of Method*. New York: Columbia University Press.

Cavan, Sheri. 1966. *Liquor License*. Chicago: Aldine.

Cicourel, Aaron V. and John Kitsuse. 1963. *The Educational Decision-Makers*. Indianapolis: Bobbs–Merrill.

Cicourel, Aaron V. 1968. *The Social Organization of Juvenile Justice*. New York: Wiley.

Cohen, Wilber J. 1968. "Independent Practitioners Under Medicare," submitted to Congress December 28.

Consumer Federation of America. 1970. "Statement of Resolutions: Concerning Chiropractic, Adopted at Annual Meeting, August 29.

Denzin, Norman K. 1970. *The Research Act*. Chicago: Aldine.

Dintenfass, Julius. 1970 (rev. ed.). *Chiropractic: A Modern Way to Health*. New York: Pyramid Books.

Douglas, Jack D. 1970. *Observations of Deviance*. New York: Random House.

———. 1971. *American Social Order*. New York: Free Press.

Duster, Troy. 1970. *The Legislation of Morality*. New York: Free Press.

Dye, A. Augustus. 1939. *The Evolution of Chiropractic: Its Discovery and Development*. Philadelphia: privately published.

Erikson, Kai T. 1964. "Notes on the Sociology of Deviance," in Howard S. Becker (ed.), *The Other Side: Perspectives on Deviance*. New York: Free Press.

———. 1966. *Wayward Puritans: A Study in the Sociology of Deviance*. New York: Wiley.

———. 1968. "Patient Role and Social Uncertainty," in Earl Rubington and Martin S. Weinberg (eds.), *Deviance: The Interactionist Perspective*. London: Macmillan, pp. 337–342.

Fineberg, Henry I. 1968. "Quackery in Review," paper presented at the Fourth National Congress on Health Quackery, Chicago, Illinois, sponsored by the American Medical Association and the National Health Council.

Freidson, E. 1965. "Disability as Social Deviance," in Marvin B. Sussman (ed.), *Sociology and Rehabilitation*. Washington: American Sociological Association.

Glaser, Barney G. and Anselm L. Strauss. 1964. "Awareness Contexts and Social Interaction," *American Sociological Review*, 29 (October): 669–679.

Goode, Erich. 1969. "Marijuana and the Politics of Reality," *Journal of Health and Social Behavior*, 10 (2) (June): 83–94.

Goffman, Irving. 1959. *The Presentation of Self in Everyday Life*. New York: Doubleday.

———. 1961. *Encounters: Two Studies in the Sociology of Interaction*. Indianapolis: Bobbs–Merrill.

———. 1963. *Behavior in Public Places*. New York: Free Press.

———. 1967. *Strategic Interaction*. Philadelphia: University of Philadelphia.

———. 1971. *Relations in Public: Microstudies in the Public Order*. New York: Basic Books.

Grim, R. W. 1972. *Chiropractic Could Save Your Life*. Louisville, Ky.: United Christian Printing Co.

Gump, Paul V. 1971. "The Behavior Setting: A Promising Unit for Environmental Designers," *Landscape Architecture*, 61 (January): 130–134.

Hoffer, Eric. 1951. *The True Believer*. New York: Harper.

Hollingshead, A. B. and Frederick C. Redlich. 1958. *Social Class and Mental Illness*. New York: Wiley.

International Chiropractic Association. *Confidential Legal Protection Handbook*. Indianapolis: International Chiropractors Insurance Company.

Leis, Gordon Leroy. 1971. *The Professionalization of Chiropractic*. Unpublished doctoral dissertation. State University of New York at Buffalo.

Lemert, Edwin M. 1967. *Human Deviance, Social Problems, and Social Control*. Englewood Cliffs, N.J.: Prentice–Hall.

Lieban, Richard W. 1966. "Sorcery, Illness, and Social Control in a Philippine Municipality," in W. R. Scott and E. H. Volkart (eds.), *Medical Care: Readings in the Sociology of Medical Institutions*. New York: Wiley, pp. 222–232.

Lindesmith, Alfred R. and Anselm L. Strauss. 1968. *Social Psychology*. New York: Holt.

Lofland, J. 1966. *Doomsday Cult: A Study of Conversion, Proselytization and Maintenance of Faith*. Englewood Cliffs, N.J.: Prentice–Hall.

MacCannel, Dean. 1973. "Staged Authenticity: Arrangements of Social Space in Tourist Settings," *American Journal of Sociology*, 79 (3): 589–603.

McCorkle, Thomas, 1961. "Chiropractic: A Deviant Theory of Disease and Treatment in Contemporary Western Culture," *Human Organization*, 20 (1): 46–62.

Matza, David. 1969. *Becoming Deviant*. Englewood Cliffs, N.J.: Prentice-Hall.

Mead, George Herbert. 1932. *Philosophy of the Present* (Merritt H. Moore, ed.). Chicago: Open Court.

————. 1934. *Mind, Self, and Society* (ed. Charles W. Morris). Chicago: University of Chicago Press.

————. 1936. *Movements of Thought in the Nineteenth Century.* Chicago: University of Chicago Press.

Mead, George Herbert. 1938. *The Philosophy of the Act* (Charles W. Morris, ed.). Chicago: University of Chicago Press.

Meltzer, Bernard N. 1964. *The Social Psychology of George Herbert Mead.* Center for Sociological Research: Western Michigan University Press.

Merton, Robert K. 1957. *Social Theory and Social Structure.* New York: The Free Press of Glencoe.

Miller, Delbert C. 1963. "Town and Gown: The Power Structure of a University Town," *American Journal of Sociology,* 68 (4) (January).

Mills, Donald L. 1966. *Study of Chiropractors, Osteopaths and Naturopaths in Canada.* Ottawa: Queen's Printer.

Natanson, Maurice. 1962. *Literature, Philosophy and the Social Sciences.* The Hague: Martinus Nijhoff.

Palmer, Daniel David. 1910. *The Chiropractor's Adjuster: A Textbook of the Science, Art, and Philosophy of Chiropractic for Students and Practitioners.* Portland, Ore.: Portland Printing House Co.

Parker, James W. 1965. *Years of Articles on Practice Building and Office Procedure.* Fort Worth, Tex.: privately printed by SHARE International.

Roebuck, Julian B. and Bruce Hunter. 1970. "Medical Quackery as Deviant Behavior," *Criminology,* 8 (1): 46–62.

————. 1972. "The Awareness of Health-Care Quackery as Deviant Behavior," *Journal of Health and Social Behavior,* 13 (June): 162–166.

Roebuck, Julian B. and Wolf Frese. *The After-Hours Club: Ethnography of an Unserious Behavior Setting* (forthcoming).

Rubington, Earl and Martin S. Weinberg. 1968. *Deviance: The Interactionist Perspective.* London: Macmillan.

————. 1971. *The Study of Social Problems.* New York: Oxford University Press.

Scheff, T. J. with the assistance of D. M. Culver. 1964. "The Societal Reaction to Deviance: Ascriptive Elements in the Psychiatric Screening of Mental Patients in a Midwestern State," *Social Problems,* 16 (Spring): 401–413.

Scheff, Thomas J. 1968. "Negotiating Reality: Notes on Power in the Assessment of Responsibility," *Social Problems*, 16 (Summer): 3–17.

Schervish, Paul G. 1973. "The Labeling Perspective: Its Bias and Potential in the Study of Political Deviance," *The American Sociologist*, 8 (May): 47–57.

Schmitt, Madeline H. 1974. "Who Goes to Chiropractors: Descriptive Data on a Sample of Medicaid Chiropractic Utilizers in the Buffalo, New York Region." Working paper submitted to the American Sociological Association, August 27, Montreal, Canada.

Schur, Edwin M. 1965. *Crimes Without Victims*. Englewood Cliffs, N.J.: Prentice–Hall.

———. 1971. *Labeling Deviant Behavior*. New York: Harper.

Schutz, Alfred. 1962. *Collected Papers, I*. The Hague: Martinus Nijoff.

Scofield, Arthur G. 1968. *Chiropractic: The Science of Specific Spinal Adjustment*. London: Thorsons.

Scott, W. R. and E. H. Volkart (eds.). 1966. *Medical Care: Readings in the Sociology of Medical Institutions*. New York: Wiley.

Senior Citizen News. January, 1969. Washington, D.C.: National Council of Senior Citizens, Inc.

Sims, L. B. 1972. "The Birth of Dynamic Essential," *Today's Chiropractic*, 1 (1) (January–February): 10.

Stephenson, Ralph W. 1948. *Chiropractic Textbook*. Davenport, Iowa: The Palmer School of Chiropractic.

Χ Sternberg, David. 1969. *Boys in Plight: A Case Study of Chiropractic Students Confronting a Medically-Oriented Society*. Unpublished doctoral dissertation, New York University.

Sussman, Marvin B. 1965. *Sociology and Rehabilitation*. Washington: American Sociological Association.

Sykes, Gresham M. and David Matza. 1957. "Techniques of Neutralization: A Theory of Delinquency," *American Sociological Review*, 22 (December): 664–670.

Thomas, W. I. 1972. *The Unadjusted Girl*. Boston: Little, Brown.

Turk, A. T. 1966. "Conflict and Criminality," *American Sociological Review*, 31 (June): 338–352.

Turner, Chittenden. 1931. *The Rise of Chiropractic*. Los Angeles: Power.

Turner, Jonathan H. 1974. *The Structure of Sociological Theory*. Homewood, Ill.: Dorsey.

Wardwell, Walter I. 1951. "Social Strain and Social Adjustment in the Marginal Role of the Chiropractor." Doctoral dissertation, Harvard University, Department of Social Relations.

————. 1952. "A Marginal Professional Role: The Chiropractor," *Social Forces*, 30: 339–348.

————. 1955. "Reduction of Strain in a Marginal Social Role," *American Journal of Sociology*, 61 (July): 16–25.

Webb, Eugene J. 1966. *Unobtrusive Measures: Nonreactive Research in the Social Sciences*. Chicago. Rand–McNally.

Williams, Sid E. 1973. Advertisement in *Today's Chiropractic*, 2 (3) (June–July): 24.

Zimmerman, Don H. and Melvin Polner. 1970. "The Everyday World as a Phenomenon," in Jack D. Douglas (ed.), *Understanding Everyday Life*. Chicago: Aldine, pp. 80–103.

Index

162 Index